New Ideas in Therapy

Recent Titles in
Contributions in Psychology

Personality, Power, and Authority: A View from the Behavioral Sciences
Leonard W. Doob

Interactive Counseling
B. Mark Schoenberg and Charles F. Preston, editors

Assessing Sex Bias in Testing: A Review of the Issues and Evaluations of 74
Psychological and Educational Tests
Paula Selkow

Position and the Nature of Personhood: An Approach to the Understanding of Persons
Larry Cochran

Ecological Beliefs and Behaviors: Assessment and Change
David B. Gray in collaboration with Richard J. Borden and Russell H. Weigel

Sexuality: New Perspectives
Zira DeFries, Richard C. Friedman, and Ruth Corn, editors

Portrait and Story: Dramaturgical Approach to the Study of Persons
Larry Cochran

The Meaning of Grief: A Dramaturgical Approach to Understanding Emotion
Larry Cochran and Emily Claspell

NEW IDEAS IN THERAPY

INTRODUCTION TO AN INTERDISCIPLINARY APPROACH

EDITED BY
Douglas H. Ruben
AND
Dennis J. Delprato

CONTRIBUTIONS IN PSYCHOLOGY, NUMBER 10
GREENWOOD PRESS
NEW YORK • WESTPORT, CONNECTICUT • LONDON

Library of Congress Cataloging-in-Publication Data

New ideas in therapy.

(Contributions in psychology, ISSN 0736-2714 ;
no. 10)

Includes bibliographies and index.

1. Behavior therapy. 2. Medicine and psychology.
I. Ruben, Douglas H. II. Delprato, Dennis J.
III. Series. [DNLM: 1. Behavior Therapy. 2. Behavioral
Medicine. W1 C0778NHH no.10 / WM 425 N5323]
RC489.B4N494   1987   616.89′142   86-31922
ISBN 0-313-24845-1   (lib. bdg. : alk. paper)

Library of Congress Catalog Card Number: 86-31922
ISBN: 0-313-24845-1
ISSN: 0736-2714

First published in 1987

Greenwood Press, Inc.
88 Post Road West, Westport, Connecticut 06881

Printed in the United States of America

The paper used in this book complies with the
Permanent Paper Standard issued by the National
Information Standards Organization (Z39.48-1984).

10   9   8   7   6   5   4   3   2   1

To the Memory of
OBSERVER

who revealed the events of behavior that were
obscured for centuries

Contents

Preface   ix

Part I. Foundations of the New Therapy

1. What Qualifies Interbehavioral Psychology as an Approach
   to Treatment?
   J. R. Kantor   3

2. Theory versus Practice?
   N. H. Pronko   9

3. From the Classroom to the Field and Back
   Paul R. Fuller   23

Part II. Methods

4. The Interbehavioral Approach to Psychopathology
   Robert W. Lundin   37

5. An Interbehavioral Approach to Clinical Child Psychology:
   Toward an Understanding of Troubled Families
   Robert G. Wahler and Della M. Hann   53

6. Toward an Interbehavioral Medicine
   F. Dudley McGlynn, Edwin W. Cook III, and Paul E.
   Greenbaum   79

7. Q Methodology: Interbehavioral and Quantum Theoretical
   Connections in Clinical Psychology
   William Stephenson   95

8. Assumptions about Teaching Assertiveness: Training the
   Person or Behavior?
   Douglas H. Ruben and Marilyn J. Ruben   107

9. Multidisciplinary Approach to Obesity and Risk-Factor
   Management
   Dallas W. Stevenson and Michael J. Hemingway   119

10. Interbehavioral Perspectives on Legal Deviance: Some
    Considerations of Context
    Edward K. Morris, Lisa M. Johnson, Lynda K. Powell,
    and James T. Todd   137

11. An Interbehavioral Perspective on Parent Training for
    Families of Developmentally Delayed Children
    Lynne A. Daurelle, James J. Fox, William E. MacLean,
    Jr., and Ann P. Kaiser   159

12. Community-Based Psychological Services for
    Developmentally Retarded Persons
    Mary Ann Scafasci   179

13. Public Policy Research from a Field-Theory Perspective
    Donna M. Cone   191

14. Value of "New Ideas"
    Douglas H. Ruben and Dennis J. Delprato   209

Index   213

About the Editors and Contributors   221

Preface

One might expect that fresh ideas would be commonplace in philosophy, basic science, and clinical science. Yet the so-called fresh ideas of the last decade all too frequently were resuscitated, refurbished, and recycled versions of the same well-worn myths and folklore. This was especially the case with views of human behavior. Attempts by behavioral science to revolutionize thinking of human behavior represented perhaps the most visible advancements in clinical psychology. The field made noteworthy strides in technology that stimulated new approaches to treatments for a number of traditional psychiatric disorders (for example, anxiety, addiction, obsessive-compulsions). As a result, treatment methods flooded the practitioner and marketplace, hurriedly replacing some traditional therapies, and thus created overambitious expectations of clinically relevant outcomes. Interest in behavioral clinical therapy exploded during the 1960s, reaching a peak by the early 1970s. Consequently the technology of behavior entered the clinical field, encouraging extensive research in psychology as a natural science.

Now, a decade later, it seems doubtful whether behavioral therapy will reach its goal of becoming a natural science. Modern behavioral therapies are so thoroughly committed to the perception of events in lineal cause-effect terms, as lawful, and as independent versus dependent variables that they overlook the obvious. Namely, simply because there are lawful relationships between phenomena does not mean that such relationships will always yield a definite or single cause. As objective psychologists, practitioners must describe clinical events in terms of multiple causes. To do this, psychology must broaden its scope to an integrated-field or systems approach that encompasses multiple causes, multiple relationships, and greater awareness of interdisciplinary study.

In this book we present a new account of therapy that takes field theory out of its theoretical shell and articulates the value of this approach for directly dealing with pressing concerns of clinical psychology. We have been influenced especially by J. R. Kantor (1888–1984), the founder of interbehaviorism whose basic assertion was the need for a behavioral system free of simple causal explanations. Kantor's alternative, and the inspiration for these chapters, was an interdisciplinary therapy. Factors of therapeutic interest should include but not be confined to traditional matters of thought, feeling, and performance; interbehaviorally, factors must also include historical, biological, social, domestic, economical, educational, vocational, and other directly confrontable events in the individual's life conditions.

This book is arranged into two sections with the interdisciplinary focus in mind. Each section avoids the generalized claim that a technology of cause and effect, of total prediction, can solve the problems of human life and society. Sections replace the illusion that instrument and measurement alone are necessary for objective scientific analysis. To this extent, each chapter first familiarizes the reader with what field theory—interbehaviorism—can do for clinical or general therapeutic interventions. In elaborating the analysis, we then redefine a recurrent or classic clinical problem from an interbehavioral perspective with applications in research and practice.

In Section 1, "Foundations of the New Therapy," attention is drawn to Kantor's unique system of human behavior of broadening orthodox learning theory toward a fuller concept of organismic interaction. We are proud to have what may be the last written work by J. R. Kantor prior to his death in 1984. His chapter, originally planned as a preface, introduces the theme of the book. N. H. Pronko's chapter clarifies the parts of Kantor's system found to be of greatest value in clinical application. Paul R. Fuller, author of the first published study of operant human conditioning, then retraces the impact of his own interbehavioral uses as teacher, consultant in the aerospace program, and clinician.

What is fundamental for Kantor and for his followers is that field theory presents a science of application. Section II, "Methods," addresses the variety of disciplines encountered in the interbehavioral network. It provides ten innovative perspectives on the field approaches to treatment. First Robert W. Lundin lays the groundwork for the interbehavioral "diagnosis" of behavior. He defines categorically Kantor's different profiles of personality within an integrated-field system. Diagnosis is expanded in the research by Robert G. Wahler and Della M. Hahn on the treatment for troubled families, closely scrutinized regarding parent-child interventions. This direction continues in the medical field as behavioral medicine attends to the interaction of biological psychological, and social variables. F. Dudley McGlynn, Edwin Cook III, and Paul E. Greenbaum propose principles for reshaping the focus of this institution.

William Stephenson's Q methodology supplies the innovation lacking in most alternatives to lineal cause-effect psychology. He defends the need for subjectivity as principal ingredient in a scientific method, as quantitatively acceptable as quantum theory. The chapters by Douglas H. Ruben and Marilyn J. Ruben and by Dallas W. Stevenson and Michael J. Hemingway directly upset the balance of tradition in conditioning theory. Ruben and Ruben, looking at assertiveness training, criticize the fallibility of generalization theory and then offer a more naturalistic conception of the learning process. Stevenson and Hemingway summarize data of their successful treatment phases in the comprehensive treatment of obesity.

Where it is orthodox in conditioning therapies to reduce larger systems to smaller units, in field theory it is heterodox. Chapters 10 through 13 are perhaps the first presentation of learning theory applied on a molar or integrated-field scale. The context of analysis deliberately remains a combination of individual and cultural events, not as separate entities, but as interdependent factions of the total setting. Edward K. Morris, Lisa M. Johnson, Lynda K. Powell, and James T. Todd, summarize their current research on the connection between socioeconomic and individual contingencies and the predisposition to deviance as a function of the legal system. Systems as a self-contained influence upon behavior is again seen in most parent-training courses. Lynne A. Daurelle, Ann P. Kaiser, and James J. Fox first review the pitfalls in theory and design of behavioral parent-training approaches; they then argue for an ecobehavioral (interbehavioral) method to extend programming in needed clinical areas.

Chapters by Mary Ann Scafasci and Donna M. Cone point out that being a specialist in so common a discipline as developmental disabilities does not guarantee objective and effective program implementation. Scafasci views the community mental health system as a product of culturalization; in her chapter she is acutely alert to many methodological mistakes. Such mistakes include when all treatment focuses on changing client behavior rather than on staff behavior as well. Cone's chief concern deals with the unused channel of authority that administrators in policy-making roles should recognize to weigh fully the benefits and risks of potential events. Into this position Cone inserts Kantor's view of culturalization as a collection of variables—historical, economic, social, religious—that all abide by the canons of science.

In the work of field theory, then, it is not enough simply to say clinical psychology invites a broader, more open outlook on human nature. Where Watson's plan was to explain behavior as reflex conditioning and Skinner's plan was to stress behavior as contingency-controlled, the interbehaviorist is most anxious to state laws of behavior as inherent in continuous interactions. The final chapter, ''Value of 'New Ideas' '' brings into focus the conclusion that by viewing clinical problems as transactional rather than as isolated phenomena the practice of psychotherapy encourages a more integrated discipline. To this end the editors hope the present work will stimulate continued development of clinical implications of the field perspective, as well as the much needed empirical evaluations of their efficacy.

_____ *Part I*

Foundations of the New Therapy

What Qualifies Interbehavioral Psychology as an Approach to Treatment?

J. R. Kantor

Among the most basic assumptions of the interbehavioral point of view is that to be effective in any sort of professional practice it is necessary to base one's efforts upon authentic scientific foundations. Engineers must be equipped with the necessary orientation in physics, chemistry, and geology. No physician can be highly rated who is not well prepared in the various branches of biology, such as anatomy, physiology, embryology, and bacteriology. Similarly, psychological clinicians cannot be capable or successful without competence in scientific psychology. It is a basic hypothesis of the present volume that interbehavioral psychology is an effective foundation for clinical applications. Success in the amelioration or radical improvement of deviant or unsatisfactory behavior may be expected by the application of interbehavioral principles.

What qualifies interbehavioral psychology for treating problems of unusual or unadaptable behavior, whether overreactions, inhibitions, or simply unsuitable responses in specific circumstances, is its derivation from *actual observations of psychological events* rather than from historical and transcendental doctrines. Interbehavioral psychology departs radically from traditional views which mythically subdivide organisms and persons into biological structures coordinated with transcendent souls, minds, or other psychic processes. In the following paragraphs are described some aspects of interbehavioral psychology favorable for clinical application.

Interbehavioral Psychology As a Natural Science

Like all authentic sciences, interbehavioral psychology consists of the unhampered analytic investigation of the interbehavior of particular organisms and the conditions under which the activities occur. In all cases, the observed interactions constitute the data or events of the particular science. Scientific events invariably comprise systems or fields. Each science is characterized by its specific type of data and the particular methods and apparatus required for understanding the events under investigation. The data of astronomy consist of the interbehavior of planets and galaxies. Physics studies action or energies as centered in various objects; chemistry investigates the interactions of numerous reagents and compounds under specific conditions of temperature, pressure, and catalysis. The data of such sciences are inorganic.

The particular psychological fields are classified as organismic and consist of a minimum of three components: (a) an organism which interacts with (b) other organisms, objects, and events under (c) definite auspices or setting factors. Before describing the details of the psychological field components, three general outstanding characteristics of psychological fields should be indicated.

Definite field origins. Psychological events as the actions of specific organisms can be precisely dated as originating in the life cycle of biological individuals. Psychological events originate a short time before birth and end with the demise of the organism concerned.

Psychological events are adaptations. To a great extent, psychological events are complex continuations of bioecological adaptations to simple and complex surroundings. Such contacts with the surroundings, in conjunction with various criteria, are denominated normal or abnormal. Suitable interbehaviors may be undeveloped, in decline, or absent.

Individual evolution. Another outstanding aspect of interbehavioral psychology is the individualistic evolution of performances and traits as organisms mature and maintain their physiological growth and vigor. Through contacts with particular items of their ambience, particular organisms develop their complex activities describable as affective, effective, linguistic, opinions, rationality, irrationality, and so on. We turn now to a brief presentation of the three primary components of psychological fields.

The Psychological Personality

Though human organisms are and always remain biological individuals—in short, animals—they belong to a species so advanced in evolution as to be able to create and maintain cultural institutions generally denominated by civilizations. Contact with the civilizational ambience greatly multiplies the nature and complexity of psychological events. Individuals thus are converted from ordinary hominids to personalities. This signifies that organisms not only interbehave with the specificities of nature—the earth, climate, atmosphere—but must also *interbehave* with things and events in numerous situations of a social, industrial, political, economic, moral, scientific, and aesthetic nature. In each situation, the person develops ways of acting in reciprocity with the development of functions by ambient things and events. The development of the organism now will consist of building up cultural interbehavior such as language, religious beliefs, moral practices, and other traits pertaining to certain civilizations. The auspices or ambience may be placed in a maturational hierarchy, the first stage of which consists of mother-child relationships. Later stages consist of interactions with family, playmates, school, community, and vocational situations. The actual interrelationships with the environment will result in the evolution of a unique personality.

In reciprocal correspondence with specific ambient things and circumstances, individuals build up responses and traits which may be represented in hierarchical order. In the earliest stages of maturation, organisms develop the elementary organic adjustments to physiological functions and infantile care. Then in succession are developed the rudimentary interbehaviors with parents or caretakers. Early on, speech and language behavior characterize the cultural evolution of human traits. Complete maturity traits include polite or impolite manners, vocational enterprise and expertise, docility, criminality, femininity, masculinity, homosexuality, conventionality and rebelliousness. In general, each individual growing up in a unique set of ambient conditions will become a unique personality subject to changes with environmental circumstances.

Personality evolution observed. Since personality evolution is a naturalistic process, it can be observed in the development of neonates. Human neonates begin as mere human evolutes. They are completely bereft of innate natures or propensities to perform psychological responses. Psychological actions and traits arise through processes of acquisition, learning, and education. These processes are basically interbehavioral adaptations to the things, persons, and events that invariably surround neonates.

For the most part, personality evolution is casual and unguided, though every family, group, or community sets up formal educational systems to influence particular types of development. Parents in cooperation with various cultural agencies will have ready blueprints for the way in which their children should behave. In compound cultures there are the notable "three R's," but for the most part, as soon as the young person can manage to do so, he or she develops on his or her own. That is, the contacts with stimulus objects, whether persons or things, are casual and the development lacks close and directed supervision. Another division of the educational process is between communal and personal traits. The communal traits of the developing organism are directed to the maintenance of certain cultural institutions, such as dialect, religion, and morality. The personal traits of education may be regarded as the basic matrix of individual differences. It is this aspect of development that results in so-called proper or improper, conforming or deviant, desirable or undesirable behavior. The undesirable behavior is the source for clinical intervention, for observation, diagnosis, and therapy.

Idiosyncratic aspects of personality evolution. Each person is a member of many human groups and each group, whether societal, political, religious, industrial, or economic, atomizes into still smaller units. Thus arise the multiplicity and intensity of individual differences. No two persons are exactly alike.

Aside from the obvious personality differences between each person's unique combination of cultural differences, there are the idiosyncratic traits in which each person develops traits that only he or she displays. Such are the unique capacities for inventions, musical composition, mathematical discovery, and other behaviors that make each person unlike any other. Such idiosyncratic traits attract the approval or disapproval of others, thereby becoming a subject of interest to clinical workers.

Stimulus Objects and Functions

The second invariable element of psychological fields consists of objects—persons, things, and circumstances. It is important to note that stimulus objects always operate on the basis of functions that are acquired through historical contacts with organisms. Each object or person acquires one or many functions. These functions pertain to use, like, dislike, ownership, and so on.

Persons take on many functions, including being liked or disliked, being pleasant or unpleasant, being clever or stupid, or being helpful or indifferent. Similarly, objects take on a variety of functions. Tables are objects on which to place things, as chairs are objects for sitting. Particular foods do or do not become good to taste or entirely inedible. In general, there are developed an infinite number of discriminative functions. Many correlate with reactions of fear and loathing, loving or hating, and numerous other affective reactions.

Auspices or Setting Factors

Since psychological organisms are at the same time organismic and inorganic entities, they and their behaviors are subject to the same conditions as the events of biology, physics, and chemistry. But in addition, psychological fields are characterized by unique circumstances. Things and persons through interbehavior with ambient objects develop functions that make psychological fields different from objects belonging to physics and biology. Response functions of organisms correlate with functions of objects established through prior interbehaviors.

Linguistic Evolution as Model of Scientific Psychology

To follow through the infantile and later development of speech and language offers an excellent model for psychological evolution. There is only one stipulation: to observe that speech is one of many types of adaptation to particular ambient circumstances. It is customary to associate speaking and the further outgrowth of language behavior with infantile vocalization. But the relationship is certainly a very remote one. The production of vocal noises basically is no more related to speech than the earliest walking behavior is a basis for going to a particular school or church. There is not yet present at this vocalization stage any circumstances for human intercourse.

As maturation proceeds, the child becomes surrounded with persons, things, and circumstances that lead to the performance of many language adjustments. Speech will develop with direct relation to the general circumstances of daily living. Comments will be made about usual or unusual happenings. Questions will be asked and answered, and various general dialogues will take place.

The language evolution model just presented not only marks the specific stages of personality development but also indicates the striking deviation of interbehavioral psychology from the conventional interpretation of speech as word utterances coupled with psychic meanings. To regard speech as verbal entities is clearly only a heritage from the time when complex linguistic adaptations were treated as things with only exegetical functions as in the interpretations of sacred textual materials.

Interbehavioral Psychology in Clinical Application

The services that a scientific psychology can offer to the work in the clinical field are many. To begin with, there are the advantages of a naturalistic approach to the problems encountered. Since clinical work concerns complaints about interbehavior, the clinician can concentrate upon the activities of integral individuals and reject guidance from traditional theoretical abstractions. He or she need not confound diagnoses and treatments with notions of internal mental states or imaginary brains, nor seek causes in nonexistent heredity.

Because psychological complaints cover an immense range, problems of normality, abnormality, deviations, or declines can be localized in the personality, in ambient conditions, and in setting factors, and then appropriately treated. Many of the complaints originate in some lack of continuity of field components. It is extremely helpful for clinical practitioners to be able to analyze complaints on a sound basis; for example, to become aware of types of complaints and their severity.

Type of complaint. In general, clinical complaints are problems of maladaptation. Behavior may be insufficient or too intense; it may affect mainly the patient, or it may affect other persons and even entire communities.

Severity of complaints. Clinical assessments are greatly influenced by the severity or intensity of the complaint or unsatisfactory situation. The deviation, loss, or decline may affect only one or a few behavior segments, or it may involve the entire personality of the patient. Again, malfunctioning may be considered as simply unusual, unadaptable, or thoroughly pathological.

Behavior may be assessed as unusual because of a mere individual difference. A child may persist in doing something that is inconvenient or undesirable. The behavior complained of may be temporary or long-lasting. But it is mildly noticeable.

Unadaptable behavior is such as to indicate a failure of orderly living. Fairly severe examples are deficiencies in learning or in social behavior conformities. Individuals may perform behavior troublesome to the family, police, and other community officials.

Pathological behaviors mark extreme personality deviations. They point to individuals who are the most serious and most troublesome. They deviate most extremely from the so-called normal personalities in their various retardations. The most serious lack the capacity to take care of themselves or develop behavior inimical to their own well-being and the safety of others.

Interbehavioral psychology may be expected to add effectively to the diagnostic analysis and the interventions of clinical practice. In addition, interbehavioral psychology as a scientific discipline may also throw light on the general problem of professional practice.

Clinical psychology and medical practice. With the burgeoning of clinical psychology as a professional branch of psychology, questions have arisen as to who should direct the analysis and treatment of behavior deviants: a psychologist or a physician? Originally, custom and law favored the latter even though it is more often the case that the psychologist is better qualified to deal with psychological problems. No doubt this situation stems from the fact that human behavior involves ecological, psychological, and sociological factors.

Although the central clinical factors are psychological, they may involve physiological problems, and thus indicate cooperative arrangements with a competent physician. Additionally, there is the claim that the psychiatrist should be the therapist in cases of behavior disorders and disturbances of societal equilibrium.

However, there are many patients who, because of birth deformities or injurious accidents, are unable to develop and perform psychological activities. But there is a great difference between deviant behavior and the destruction of biological structures and functions of individuals.

Always there remains the question of the psychological competence of practitioners. It is a rare experience to find a psychiatrist who has rejected the venerable dualism of mind and body. With an interbehavioral psychology background, both the analysis of abnormal behavior and the problems of psychology and medical practice can be cleared up.

Theory versus Practice?   **2**

N. H. Pronko

A careful reading of the *Journal of Clinical Psychology* for 1982 and 1983 reveals an assiduous busyness on the part of clinical practitioners. It is as if they were goaded into action by the stern command "Don't just stand there. Do something!" The succession of articles displays a profusion of interests. There are articles on psychodynamics and psychopathology. There are pieces on the outcome of treatment variables. For example, on *x* personality test, performance of Group A (depressed) is compared with the performance of Group B (non-depressed), or Group A's performance on Test A is compared with its performance on Test B. Correlation, factor analysis, and other statistical measures reign supreme. In an "Invited Editorial," M. Lorr (1982) recommends the use of such sophisticated multivariate procedures as cluster analytic techniques and ordination.

One should not presume to tell the researchers in the population reviewed above how to go about their business of manipulating the variables of interest to them. However, one looks in vain for a recognition of the postulates, assumptions, and presuppositions that guide their research, despite the fact that certain studies clearly have either a psychoanalytic, a phenomenological, or a cognitive flavor. It appears that J. H. Woodger's (1929) commentary on his own field of biology is just as applicable to the work under review:

Nothing is more striking in this science than the contrast between the brilliant skill, ingenuity and care bestowed upon observation and experiment, and the almost complete neglect of caution in regard to the definition and use of the concepts in terms of which its results are expressed. (p. 3)

Assuming the validity of Woodger's observation, one wants to reverse the injuction above to read: "Don't just do something. Stand there a while and think about what you're going to do and what it is that you've done after you've done it." In other words, what is missing is *theory* both as a guide to research and as an explanation of it. It seems appropriate to conclude this brief assessment of clinical work with Leonardo da Vinci's perceptive observation: "Those who fall in love with practice without science are like a sailor who enters a ship without a helm or a compass, and who never can be certain whither he is going" (quoted by Johnston & Pennypacker, 1980). The missing "helm" or "compass" to which da Vinci refers is an appropriate metaphor for the paradigm.

This chapter takes as its focus da Vinci's observation that assumptions guiding theory and practice are essential in clinical psychology. We examine how scientific observation is an unavoidably theory-laden enterprise. This leads to a survey of paradigms extant in contemporary psychology and whether they can all be categorized as self-actional, interactional, or transactional. Next, we explore the possibility of doing clinical work either without a guiding theory or under one or another of the traditional paradigms. Rejecting both of the alternatives, we try to show their shortcomings and propose an interbehavioral approach as a profitable substitute.

Concerning Paradigms

Today, scientists, particularly social scientists, show an increasing sensitivity to the paradigms or models that govern their research. Much of the credit for this movement must be attributed to T. S. Kuhn's (1970) widely read book *The Structure of Scientific Revolutions*. Kuhn views science not as a disembodied, impersonal entity but as the activity of a social/psychological group or scientific community. The ongoing activity of the group members has produced certain achievements which provide models for scientific research. Adherents are attracted to the group and become committed to the group and continue the traditional program. They share the paradigms of their predecessors (i.e., the theories, beliefs, values, attitudes, applications, instrumentation), read the same literature, undergo the same training, and come out as psychological clones of their mentors. More interesting still is the fact that, despite the advocacy of a shared paradigm as a guide for research, its followers do not feel the need to produce "a full interpretation or rationalization of it" (Kuhn, 1970, p. 44). They stick to the model in an unwitting or tacit sense with the conviction that the paradigm accounts successfully for the observations and experiments which it subsumes.

Further development . . . ordinarily calls for the construction of elaborate equipment, the development of an esoteric vocabulary and skills, and a refinement of concepts that increasingly lessens their resemblance to their usual common-sense prototypes. That professionalization leads, on the one hand, *to an immense restriction of the scientist's vision and to a considerable resistance to paradigm change. The science has become increasingly rigid.* [emphasis mine] (Kuhn, 1970, p. 64)

This is "normal science." One comes away from Kuhn's penetrating analysis of scientists at work with the feeling that their paradigms exert a control on them similar to that imposed on the disciples of a monastic order.

But normal science does not continue in perpetuity. Crises occur with the advent of new discoveries and the development of new theories, neither of which fits the traditional paradigm. When confronted by anomalies, scientists have responded by devising ad hoc amendments to existing theory in order to handle the apparent anomaly. For example, if the removal of a large portion of a cerebral hemisphere does not produce a behavior deficit, why not say that the remaining hemisphere has "taken over" the function previously performed by the former? Such an amendment rescues the threatened paradigm.

When anomalies become too obvious and ad hoc adjustments lead to a blurring of the prevailing paradigm, a breakdown occurs and a new candidate for paradigm emerges. With the abandonment of the old paradigm, "the scientist's perception of his environment must be reeducated" (Kuhn, 1970, p. 112) and again, "though the world does not change with a change of paradigm, the scientist afterward works in a different world" (Kuhn, 1970, p. 121). Kuhn compares the rejection of the discarded paradigm for the new one as a "conversion experience" or a paradigm shift.

Scientific revolutions have a drastic effect on their participants. Here is the way Kuhn puts it:

It is rather as if the professional community had been suddenly transported to another planet where familiar objects are seen in a different light and are joined by unfamiliar ones as well. Of course, nothing of quite that sort does occur: there is no geographical transplantation; outside the laboratory everyday affairs usually continue as before. Nevertheless, paradigm changes do cause scientists to see the world of their research-engagement differently. In so far as their only recourse to that world is through what they see and do, we may want to say that after a revolution scientists are responding to a different world. (1970, p. 111)

To further explain the effect of a paradigm shift, Kuhn makes use of the well-known ambiguous figure as developed by the Gestalt school. For our purposes, let us take the familiar Rubin figure as an example. This geometrical form permits the actualization of two different discriminatory responses. First, you may see the goblet, but, a moment later, you see two people in silhouette staring at each other. If you continue to look at the figure, you are free to switch back and forth between the two perceptual possibilities. This is not so in the case of scientists who have been won over to the new paradigm. Their commitment to it prevents their switching back and forth between the old and new ways of seeing their data. Their reeducation has been completed and they see things only in the new way. They have a brand-new global orientation, a different worldview. We now move on to a further examination of how we see things, this time by way of N. R. Hanson's contribution to a most fundamental scientific procedure, namely, observation.

Observation

Observation appears to be the proper starting point for any scientific activity. As a starter, let us examine Figure 2.1, "The Burning Tree." What do you observe? A large tree and several smaller ones? A forest fire in the background? A discharge of lightning? A portion of a blood circulatory system, showing arteries or veins branching into capillaries? Nerve processes innervating some tissue? Actually, Figure 2.1 is an infrared aerial photo of a river delta. Now, with a shift like that involved in an ambiguous gestalt figure, do you see it as a river delta?

What is the point of this exercise? The purpose is to show that we do not see unvarnished facts. Otherwise, how could we have seen such a variety of things in the same geometrical pattern? Science students are exhorted to stick with "the facts." Make accurate observations of the so-called raw data and you cannot go wrong; they will lead you to their proper understanding. But is it not true that if our seeings were of pristine, raw "sensations" that we would see only meaningless shapes in Figure 2.1 instead of the rich variety of discriminations that that visual pattern evoked? We would have to be stricken with a total visual amnesia to be reduced to such a state. On the contrary, our little experiment demonstrates that much of our past visual experiences are brought to bear in our inspection of Figure 2.1.

We are now ready for help furnished us by N. R. Hanson's (1958) discussion of observation in his book *Patterns of Discovery*. Hanson takes the case of two microbiologists viewing an amoeba under a microscope. Although both focus on the same object and both have normal vision, they do not see the same thing. One sees it as analogous to such single cells as liver, epithelium, and so on, the only difference being that it is an independent cell and not a part of a tissue. The second microbiologist sees the amoeba as analogous to a whole animal because, like other animals, the amoeba ingests its food, digests and assimilates it. Besides, it excretes, moves around and reproduces, in these respects resembling a whole animal instead of a single cell. The important point is that their differences cannot be solved via any experiment, but such differences can determine their design of experiments. This and still other examples of different scientists looking at the same things but seeing them differently support Hanson's statement that "there's more to seeing than meets the eyeball" (1958, p. 7). The eyeball can only register physical excitation; there is no use in looking behind the eyeball for any act that might be labeled as "seeing." Why? Because it is *people* who see and not their eyes. Some psychologists would agree that when people see different things in Figure 2.1 their retinal reactions might be

Figure 2.1
What is it? A grove of trees stripped of most of their leaves? A forest fire in the background? A photo of a bolt of lightning? A portion of a blood circulatory system, with arteries or veins branching into capillaries? Nerve processes innervating some tissue? For a clue as to what this photo "really" captured, see the text.

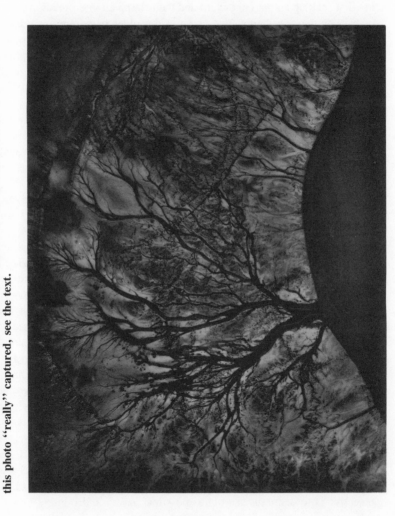

Photo by permission of Aero Service Division, Western Geophysical Company of America.

identical. However, it is the different interpretations that they put upon them that explain the differences in their discriminations.

Hanson has much to say on this point. If he were looking at the Rubin figure and, first, sees the vase, then the two faces, he would insist that he does not do two things each time—seeing and interpreting. When he shifts from one discrimination to another only seeing is involved. As Hanson states it, "one does not first soak up an optical pattern and then clamp an interpretation on it" (1958, p. 9). For the time being, and as an aside, older paradigms imagined that the alleged interpretation of sensations occurred somewhere in the brain. Hanson apprehends the force of traditional notions in determining our seeings as revealed in the following statement: "There is a sense in which seeing is a 'theory-laden' undertaking. Observation of x is shaped by prior knowledge of x" (1958, p. 19). Our language habits also play a role in shaping our seeings. One cannot improve on the following strong Hansonian metaphor. "Facts are moulded by the logical forms of the language used in talking about the facts. Perhaps these provide a 'mould' in terms of which the world coagulates for us in definite ways" (1958, p. 36). From then on, we are stuck with a rigidified view of that coagulated world.

Let us assume that a number of psychologists are observing a given psychological event. Do they all see the same thing? Probably not. A sees something, although invisible, going on inside the organism's mind which A labels consciousness. B "improves" upon A claiming an unconscious, that is, an unconscious conscious. C sees superego at war with the id on the battleground of the ego. D sees engrams and speech and smell centers. In former times, the same psychologists might have seen mental faculties such as will, memory, and attention. Why do they not see the same thing? Because everyone's seeing is "theory-laden." The dice are loaded because each has learned to see according to the paradigm acquired during training. The vocabulary that adherents learned in school provided a mold in terms of which the world coagulated for them in accordance with the paradigm espoused by each. We now turn to an inspection and analysis of the different paradigms that we find in use among psychologists.

Structuralism, functionalism, classical behaviorism, radical behaviorism, Gestalt, humanistic psychology, psychoanalysis, cognitivism, eclecticism—what a bewildering array of uncongenial schools! Nevertheless, their essential differences can be defined in a fundamental way by assigning these disparate approaches to psychology to one of three categories. These categories are derived from Bentley's (1935, 1954) and Dewey and Bentley's (1949) work. Our next objective is to define as sharply as possible Dewey and Bentley's categories of self-action, interaction, and transaction.

Self-action

A contemporary textbook of psychology (Janda & Klenke-Hamel, 1980) reads as follows: "Much of our behavior and many of our sensations and skills are governed by the nervous system. . . . The brain is a sophisticated machine for communicating, for receiving and storing information and for issuing instructions concerning all our bodily functions and mental activities'' (p. 38, 42). Here is an example par excellence of self-action. *Webster's Collegiate Dictionary* defines *self-action* as ''acting or capable of acting by itself; automatic.'' Dewey and Bentley's elaboration of the term sees self-action ''where things are viewed as acting under their own powers'' (1949, p. 108). Note that in the quotation above, the nervous system is described as ''governing'' our behavior, and many of our sensations and skills. The brain is said to be a ''sophisticated machine.''

As defined by Dewey and Bentley, Janda and Klenke-Hamel's attribution of the various managerial functions to the brain fits the notion of self-action. The implication is that there is a separate entity within the person that initiates and controls action. For some it is the brain, for others it is the mind, consciousness, the unconscious, ego, the self, instinct, talent, native IQ, genius, drive, and so on. Such innate agents, forces, or abilities allegedly reside within the organism. Karl Pearson saw through such hypothetical entities and offered the following pithy comment: ''To know requires exertion, and it is intellectually easiest to shirk effort altogether by accepting *phrases which cloak the unknown in the undefinable*'' [emphasis added] (1911, p. ix). Or as Hanson so cogently put it: ''What requires explanation cannot itself figure in the explanation'' (1958, p. 120). And, if added emphasis of this point is called for, one can hardly improve on Kuhn's declaration: ''Merely conceivable theories are not among the options open to the practicing scientist'' (1961, p. 177). If it were otherwise, then whatever explanation one might ''dream up'' would be equally acceptable.

Interaction

''Where thing is balanced against thing in causal interconnection'': this is Dewey and Bentley's (1949, p. 188) definition of interaction. With an interactional approach, ''power'' is shared with another object. We now have two variables acting upon one another as in Newton's third law of motion. Strike one billiard ball with another and you have demonstrated that action and reaction are equal and opposite. You have also exemplified interaction. What we have here are two separate things acting upon each other, sometimes in mutual or reciprocal action. Applied to psychology, the interactional approach no longer localizes behavior within the organism alone. As an example, the psychophysical experiment studied the relationship between stimulus differences and the corresponding sensory experiences. It belongs in the interactional category because it measured two things in causal interconnection. Stimulus-response psychology fits the interactional pattern when it is involved with fragments of behavior lifted out of the context of their behavioral continuity. Before leaving the topic of interaction, we should note that sometimes self-actional explanation may resemble interaction, but its acknowledgment of the stimulus is only grudging and forced. Most of the credit goes to the brain or mind and the other variable, the stimulus, is allowed the minor role of a trigger.

Transaction

In the study of behavioral data, one can treat events as unitary, or one can view them as fragments of separate entities or elements. If the second choice is made, one gets into the problem of gluing the fragments together into some kind of synthesis or organization by some external agency or "principle." The problem does not arise with the first alternative, which deals in total integrated events. Such an approach, the transactional viewpoint, developed by Dewey and Bentley (1949), starts with "unfractured observation." They never forget that whether you focus on the organism, the stimulus object, or setting factor, you are only talking about an *aspect* of the whole situation, occurrence, or field. With a transactional approach, the locus of behavior is no longer bounded by the skin of the organism. Behavior, in a metaphorical sense, "spills over" into the entire system of discernible factors that make up the situation.

A Summing Up

What is the result of our review of paradigms for psychology? To me, the most astounding finding is that the self-actional and interactional procedures together have survived for 2,000 years. While physics and astronomy have had a number of scientific revolutions, psychology has had none. For centuries, ours has been what Kuhn calls "normal science." And, if you should mention Watson's *behaviorism*, I would remind you that that was an aborted revolution and that mainstream psychology today is back at square one. If Shakespeare, dead for over 350 years, were to be resurrected, he would be unable to follow contemporary physics, astronomy, or biology. But he would feel right at home in mainstream psychology. For example, in *King Lear*, in explaining senility, Shakespeare assigned the following lines to Lear: "We are not ourselves when nature, being oppressed, commands the mind to suffer with the body." That certainly has a modern ring to it.

Theory

Confronted with the perplexing confusion of theories prevalent in contemporary psychology, the clinician may proclaim "a plague on all your houses" and attempt to carry on his work without any theoretical guidance. I know of a clinician who in total frankness confessed that he would sometimes achieve excellent results with a troubled client without being able to say, afterward, what he *had* done or *how* he had succeeded. Apparently, he had hit upon the right maneuver by pure happenstance.

What is wrong with such a bumbling procedure? What would you think of a chemist who mixed elements and compounds until they produced an explosion without being able to identify which elements and compounds had been used and in what order? Whatever your answer, it applies as well to our bumbling clinician. Hit-or-miss treatments may end in success, but they more often end in failure, a point admitted by my clinician friend. Are haphazard procedures ever commendable? Surely, there are parents who have reared happy, fulfilled, creative children without knowing a thing about psychology. How did they do it? They cannot tell you. Apparently, they *happened* to do "the right things," things that changed to be based upon sound psychological principles. Other parents unwittingly chanced to do other things, with sad consequences.

It would follow that sound psychological procedures, rather than fortuitous ones, should benefit clinicians as well as parents. This is the point at which psychological theory deserves consideration as a guide toward clinical practice in contradistinction to the preceding haphazard manner of handling people's problems. In the final analysis, if it is true that all observations are theory laden, then it follows that even those clinicians who bumble along in their clinical practice without theory are influenced in what they do by the way they have wittingly or unwittingly learned to see things. Since no one ever escapes some kind and degree of theoretical indoctrination, then we are not talking about theory versus no theory, but of valid theory versus bad theory. At this juncture, we proceed to a consideration of theory applied to clinical practice.

Working with a Theory

Assuming that our illustrative clinician should abandon the avoidance of theory, which of the psychological theories should be given tentative trial? Instead of examining the suitability of each separate school as to its handling of clinical data, we may frugally lump them all under the categories *self-action*, *interaction*, or *transaction*. Considering self-actional theories first, with their heavy emphasis on the alleged contents of the organism's skin, we are confronted with such mechanistic expressions as *"encode, read out from storage, reverberating circuits, overloaded channels, gating, pressure, flow, drainage, networks, centers,* or *cell assemblies"* (Skinner, 1969, p. 83). Besides such "physical" entities as the foregoing, we also encounter psychical creations—the mind, consciousness, id, ego, superego, mental representations, images, and so on. The compelling question of the clinician-in-search-of-a-theory at this point might well go something like this: "I work with relationships involving parent and child, teacher and pupil, husband and wife. Pray tell me how can I apply your imaginary entities, supposedly encapsulated within the organism, to the down-to-earth, persistent problems in human relations that I grapple with?" We can only imagine the self-actionist theoretician's retort.

Should our clinician-in-quest-of-help in understanding human relationships change upon an interactional type of theorist, their dialogue might run as follows: "Your simplistic S-R formulation grudgingly allows the stimulus to play a minor role in psychological events, but you still endow the brain and the mind to 'encode,' 'store,' 'process,' and 'retrieve.' I find even your latest inventions, such as your cognitivists' 'mental models of reality' too ethereal to be of any practical help to me.''

Our clinician-in-search-of-a-theory might give us in thoroughgoing frustration at this point. But if patience and persistence prevailed, further inquiry would lead to a third approach to clinical data which, in my opinion, would serve such a function adequately. This is interbehavioral theory, which we consider indirectly by way of Sullivan's (1950) theory of interpersonal relations in the hope that his approach can serve as a halfway house in our progress toward an interbehavioral framework for clinical practice.

Sullivan's View

Self-actional and interactional theories, with their chief focus on the organism, view the organism as individual, autonomous, and self-determined. But Harry Stack Sullivan did not. He rejected both mind and the individual human being as a workable notion. For him a ''person'' or ''personality'' was a myth and a delusion. Sullivan was willing for the biologist to talk about individual specimens of men, but for understanding psychological events one must realize that ''to be a person it is necessary that one live in the world of persons and personal entities, and personal organization, and so on'' (1950, p. 331):

What the personality does, which can be observed and studied only in relations between personalities or among personalities, is truly and terribly marvelous, and is human, and is the function of creatures living in indissoluble contact with the world of culture and of people. In the field, it is preposterous to talk about individuals and to go on deceiving oneself with the idea of uniqueness, of single entity, of simple, central being. (Sullivan, 1950, p. 329)

In applying his distinctive orientation to his patients, Sullivan could not see an individual suffering from ''mental disease,'' mental illness, or behavior pathology. For him, there were only disturbed interpersonal relations. Accordingly, he defined his job as the study and modification of the *relevant network of interpersonal relations* in which his patient was caught. He sought to modify such disturbed relations by entering into them and by being a part of them as a participant observer. His approach is quite different from the heavy concentration on the organism upon which other approaches rely. His use of an expanded observational base should facilitate our transition to our next topic, interbehavioral theory.

An Interbehavioral Framework for Clinical Practice

The interbehavioral approach toward such data as confront the clinician demands a radical shift in orientation. No longer is the emphasis on the autonomous organism and autonomous stimulus, whether viewed in a symmetrical or asymmetrical relationship. The traditional self-actional organism as the source and locus of psychological happenings is abandoned, as is the popular but obsolescent S-R (stimulus-response) or cause-effect formulation that necessitates somehow uniting the detached entities with which one starts by some sort of magical glue, such as "relationship." According to the interbehaviorist, the pristine observation yields only an unfractured, integrated field event. That is why the interbehaviorist asks of the traditionalist, "Why is it that even prior to any investigation you fixate on the organism and stimulus object as if they were the whole thing?"

In the interbehavioral view of psychological events, the organism and stimulus object are not neglected. Indeed, they play a nuclear role in the total event, but *only a partial aspect of the whole affair*. Furthermore, the interbehaviorist takes into account additional aspects: the medium of contact and setting factors.

Medium of contact. If you are reading a book and the lights go out, your reading comes to a halt. Why? Because a condition (light) which had permitted the organism and stimulus object to enter into a psychological relationship is absent. Air and water provide a medium of contact for auditory interactions. There are still other media of contact (Pronko, 1980, pp. 25–26), but these examples will suffice to clarify the difference between the traditional treatment of these factors and the interbehaviorist's treatment. The traditionalist handles light and air waves as stimuli which the brain or mind creates into "percepts."

Setting factors. Let us take a familiar situation. Students are performing an experiment in a chemistry laboratory. As they work, they joke with each other and they may even utter vulgarities. However, their coarse humor has no effect on the results of their chemical interactions. But imagine the consequences of transferring such a setting to the psychology laboratory where humans are engaged in a memory experiment. Jokes or other distractions could ruin such an experiment in psychology, but they do not in chemistry or physics. The crucial role played by the conditions surrounding the organism and stimulus object is provided by a case reported by Moser (1965, p. 90A), a story with a clinical flavor.

Billy was an exemplary child, but only under highly specific conditions; that is, when his father, a strict disciplinarian, was at home. As soon as his father drove off to work, Billy manifested a radical personality switch. He went berserk, tearing up his mother's evening clothes and urinating on them. He then proceeded to smash the furniture and otherwise vandalize the home. He also tore the buttons off his shirt and defecated in his pants, even though his mother liked to have him look nice.

In trying to fathom Billy's behavior, what approaches are open to the clinician? Can a study of the child's genes, brain traces, or his mental states help to solve the problem? In line with traditional theories, how would one even *begin* such inquiries? Applying an interbehavioral approach, why not try that which is directly observable—Billy's changing situation, or setting factors. The presence or absence of Billy's father is the crucial factor in Billy's behavior. In fact, we can control and predict the child's action by manipulating this single variable.

If further examples of setting factors are required, consider the specificity of conditions that surround human lovemaking or the habits that surround the elimination of body wastes. Of 1,419 college students, Williams and Degenhardt (1954) found that 14.4 percent experienced "difficulty (or impossibility) of initiating the flow of urine in the presence of others" (p. 20) even when there were stall separations. Acknowledging setting factors as a valuable source of information for the investigative clinician, we move on to a consideration of the interbehavioral history as an additional clinical tool: "He who sees things from their beginnings will have the most advantageous view of them" (Gesell, 1945, p. 1).

It seems like a reasonable assumption that Billy's behavior had an origin. Here is where Kantor's (1924, pp. 180–84) early formulation can stand us in good stead. The interbehavioral history refers to the complete psychological history of a given individual. The following quotation from Skinner (1959) harmonizes with Kantor's formulation: "We make some progress toward understanding anything when we discover how it is related to other things, especially to antecedent events" (p. 229). And so, in the faith that present events are a function of antecedent events, we delve into Billy's past, consulting teachers, pediatricians, and significant others in an attempt to unravel Billy's career as a "problem child." We cannot emphasize strongly enough that here again our procedure deals only with observables. With respect to the earlier events in Billy's interbehavioral history, while admittedly they are not *now* present, they are nevertheless *observable* and require only ingenuity leading to their discovery. The situation is comparable to that of the astronomer who failed to see either a recent eclipse or one in the dim historical past. Both events are, or were, potentially observable.

Useful and Useless Theories

The interbehavioral theory that I have sketched above is in accord with the data of Billy's case. It fits. It also yields an understanding of Billy's behavior and a procedure for dealing with it. The relationship between data and construct is analogous to a two-way street in the sense that we derive a theory from observing the data; that is one way. Then, we refer back to the data strictly *in terms of that theory*; that is the other direction. Stated otherwise, from observing the data we derive constructs of organism-stimulus object interaction, setting factors, interbehavioral history, and present events as a function of antecedent events. This easy passage back and forth between the crude datum level and the theoretical level suggests the analogy of a two-way street:

By contrast, traditional theory, dealing, as it does, with non-observable, hypothetical entities, implies a one-way street because the connection between the crude datum level and construct level (i.e., genes, hormones, brain traces or mental states) has been broken. There is no congruence between the two levels; consequently, no application. Under the circumstances, in working with people's problems, why not test the usefulness of the more recent theories such as the interbehavioral viewpoint . . .

If the results of such an application of interbehavioral type of theory would fall in line with . . . expectations, they would disprove the old notion that an insurmountable barrier separates the theoretician and the practitioner. As a physicist, Einstein never performed a laboratory experiment in his life. However, he was an honored theoretician who, nevertheless, depended on the experimentalist to confirm or negate his theories and to provide him with observational data. Similar possibilities exist in psychology if unprofitable, one-way-street theories give way to testable, two-way-street paradigms. . . . If and when such a golden age should come to pass, one in which the academician and the practitioner come together to work in a joint, cooperative enterprise, I can almost hear them affirming in unison: "Nothing is more practical than a good theory." (Pronko, 1982, p. 430)

References

Bentley, A. F. 1935. *Behavior knowledge fact*. Chicago: Principia Press.

Bentley, A. F. 1954. *Inquiry into inquiries: Essays in social theory*. Boston: Beacon Press.

Dewey, J., and A. F. Bentley. 1949. *Knowing and the known*. Boston: Beacon Press.

Gesell, A. 1945. *The embryology of behavior*. New York: Harper.

Hanson, N. R. 1958. *Patterns of discovery*. Cambridge, England: Cambridge University Press.

Janda, L. H., and K. E. Klenke-Hamel. 1980. *Psychology: Its study and uses*. New York: St. Martin's Press.

Johnston, J. M., and H. S. Pennypacker. 1980. *Strategies and tactics of human behavioral research*. Hillsdale, N.J.: Lawrence Erlbaum Associates.

Kantor, J. R. 1924. *Principles of psychology*, vol. 1. New York: Alfred A. Knopf.

Kuhn, T. S. 1961. The function of measurement in modern, physical science. *Isis* 52: 161–93.

Kuhn, T. S. 1970. *The structure of scientific revolutions*, 2nd ed. Chicago: University of Chicago Press.

Lorr, M. 1982. On the use of cluster analytic techniques. *Journal of Clinical Psychology* 38: 461–62.

Moser, D. May 1965. Screams, scraps, and love. *Life*, pp. 90A–101.

Pearson, K. 1911. *The grammar of science*, 2nd ed. London: Adam & Charles Black.

Pronko, N. H. 1980. *Psychology from the standpoint of an interbehaviorist*. Monterey, Calif.: Brooks/Cole.

Pronko, N. H. 1982. Practice versus theory? *Academic Psychology Bulletin* 4: 425–30.

Skinner, B. F. 1959. *Cumulative record*. New York: Appleton-Century-Crofts.

Skinner, B. F. 1969. *Contingencies of reinforcement*. New York: Appleton-Century-Crofts.

Sullivan, H. S. 1950. The illusion of personal individuality. *Psychiatry* 13: 317–32.

Williams, G. W., and E. T. Degenhardt. 1954. Paruresis: A survey of a disorder of
    micturition. *Journal of General Psychology* 51: 19–29.
Woodger, J. H. 1929. *Biological principles: A critical study*. New York: Kegan, Paul,
    Trench & Trubner.

3

From the Classroom to the Field and Back

Paul R. Fuller

This chapter traces an evolution of application of the data and methods of objective psychology from the standpoint of one interbehaviorist. The narrative spans four decades—a period of exciting growth for science and psychology, especially for applied psychology.

A generation or two ago, it was rare for a person to progress from undergraduate to Ph.D. majoring in psychology from the beginning. Medicine, math, engineering, and other established career choices were often made at an early age and pursued without wavering. This was not the case with psychology. Many could not spell the word when entering college, much less know what it might mean as a career. This author was no exception. Before entering the army of the United States in World War II, he was majoring in geology and minoring in physics and chemistry. Finding himself more interested in the "human condition" when he returned, he majored in government and psychology, hoping to find in psychology some basis for a sound political theory which seemed to be needed in 1945. The search continued.

Editors' note:

Fuller's chapter departs from the academic conventions of writing style and uses the first-person pronoun more than other chapters in this book. His presentation is deliberately more informal, subjective, and retrospective of personal experiences undertaken to explore the viewpoints of a field psychologist. Observations of Fuller's own adjustments as teacher, clinician, and consultant in broadening his approach to psychology classically illustrate the transition that can be expected from any behavioral practitioner who follows a similar path. In a casual style, Fuller better relates the pragmatic risks and benefits of field theory for an emotional understanding of the position.

Initial Experiences

Since most of this chapter is based on personal observations, let us switch to the first-person pronoun.

While recovering from the war in Europe and preparing for the final assault in Japan, I worked in the Rehabilitation Battalion, U.S. Army Hospital, Springfield, Missouri. We conducted group sessions for surgical patients who were undergoing nerve, bone or plastic surgery which kept them in the hospital for a long time. We worked on maintaining and stimulating "cognitive functions" while others worked on physical rehabilitation. This has been a recurring activity, including work with cancer patients and their families. In war time and other crisis situations we find ourselves trying many new activities, including some for which we have not been trained. Often innovations occur under unlikely circumstances. Fortuitous circumstances shape scientific developments more than most of us suspect or care to admit.

While at Indiana University (IU) Robert Urmston and I were involved in studying the effects of glutamic acid on test performance of intellectually impaired children. While working in the residential treatment center in southern Indiana we became acquainted with many residents other than the hundred in our study. One was what they called in those days a "vegetative idiot." The general opinion was that he and those like him had learned nothing and could not learn anything. I received permission to feed him his meals. Thus I was able through operant conditioning techniques to teach him to raise his arm to a vertical position—a completely new behavior for him. This became the first published account of the use of operant conditioning with a human subject. It was reprinted in several books and after nearly forty years requests for reprints are still received. It was an unplanned and unforeseen event which had consequences for the treatment of more than just the retarded.

Aside from exhortation, telling someone what to do, to "buck up" and the like, the psychoanalytic and the Rogerian "nondirective" approaches were predominant in the 1940s. There were some who were seeking a more scientific basis for psychotherapy in theories and knowledge of learning and conditioning. This was viewed as subversive by many of the supervising psychiatrists and psychologists of the day. The first example I encountered in the Indiana University Psychological Clinic involved a grade-school boy who had been seen for one semester by an advanced graduate student for play therapy. Diagnostically he was "antisocial."

The Antisocial Child

The approach to this child first began in the typical Rogerian, nondirective fashion. The therapist typically emerged from the sesssion splattered with modeling clay, finger paint, and the like. When the therapist introduced me and began to explain that there would be a transfer eventually to me, the boy protested and said, "What are you guys up to, what are you trying to do?" and ran from the room. After duly reflecting his feelings à la Rogers, we decided to give chase and overtook him at the "Jordan River," as the campus creek was called. After considerable conversation, two moderately large adult males convinced the boy to return to the clinic. At the earliest opportunity I proposed to the director, Dr. Beier, that I would like to move from the restrictive play therapy and permissive sessions in order to begin to shape some prosocial behavior through differential reinforcement. I was vehemently told, "You cannot treat this child the way you do your rats and pigeons or your vegetative idiot!" I was to stick to play therapy and finger painting. We had already begun to suspect what was subsequently demonstrated—*nondirective therapy is not completely nondirective*. Through facial expression, gestures, body language, "uh-huh," and other speech the therapist unintentionally or otherwise shapes the verbal and other behavior of the client. I chose to plan to do it intentionally.

I first had to determine just what the objectives were. I hoped that something more than practicum credit for a graduate student would be the result. The boy had been referred for antisocial behavior which reached a peak when he burned down a house. Much of the behavior in the therapy sessions could be classified as antisocial—throwing art materials, for example. When it appeared that he could not completely control the situation, he ran, or tried to run away. Furthermore, when one backed away from the medical or psychoanalytic model, one could see that although he displayed some destructive, antisocial behavior, he also displayed some very desirable behavior.

Another proposition was considered. If what a client does in the clinic—taking tests, playing, talking—has a relationship to other behavior, it is a two-way street, an interaction. If painting fire, blood, and violence in the clinic is related to fire-setting and violent behavior outside the clinic, why could not changes evolved in the clinic have an effect outside? If this were not the case, the usefulness of the clinical procedures were in doubt. A set of goals were determined; a menu of reinforcers (mostly social) was established and work began. We proceeded to meet in the psychology clinic and continued to use the materials in the play room, but a shaping process was instituted. When he threw or started to throw things, they were removed. When he painted less violent scenes, they were socially and at times tangibly reinforced.

Not having been told that psychologists do not make house calls, and being a graduate student and not entitled to call myself a psychologist anyway, I visited his school and home where I found much positive behavior. I enlisted the cooperation of the significant adults to recognize and strengthen it. From some time, his violent, antisocial behavior had received most of the reactions from family and school. By the end of the semester his finger paintings were peaceful and beautiful, and his antisocial behavior in the office, home, and school changed. I am sure that if he had known a word for it, he would have said that his "self-concept" had greatly improved.

Opportunities to develop and expand the application of interbehavioral psychology came through the Indiana University Traveling Speech and Hearing Clinic and a two-year internship with the Veterans Administration (VA) (1950– 52). At that time, there was little question as to the predominance of the medical doctor in hospitals and nonuniversity clinics. While it was accepted that the Ph.D. was a scholarly research degree, there was disagreement as to just what work the psychologist would be allowed to do. Research was accepted. Administration of tests was accepted generally. Some M.D.'s thought psychologists could do psychotherapy under medical supervision; some thought psychologists were the best-qualified psychotherapists and that M.D.'s could give drugs, shock treatment, physical examinations, and strictly medical practices. The official position was that the only people who could conduct therapy were medical doctors. This environment was the setting for one of the biggest emotional explosions I had seen in the field. A psychology professor maintained that neurotic behavior was learned and that psychologists were experts on learning and even had mathematical theories of learning; therefore, psychologists were qualified to treat neurosis through application of these principles of learning. This stimulated a prominent psychiatrist, previously thought to be friendly toward psychologists, to explode. There was such a chain reaction that "learn" became a dirty word, because to the psychiatrists learning meant things like Pavlovian conditioning or memorization of nonsense syllables.

In truth, it was not all that easy to apply what we knew of learning and conditioning to work in the hospital, but the IU interns became very adept at translating objective constructs into the terms and constructs of Jungian or Freudian psychoanalytic theory. We learned a lot, achieved a lot, and were complimented by supervising psychiatrists because we were "so objective."

My Ph.D. dissertation was researched in the VA hospitals where I was able to study some of the physiological and psychological effects of subshock doses of insulin. Among other facts, the primary reinforcing effects of sweetened orange juice in shaping behavior were studied, as were the increased secondary reinforcing effects of approval of the one who gives the patient the orange juice. This was also an example of a two-way interaction. It is not only what is given, but who gives it and how it is given along with other setting factors. It is small wonder that what is thought to be the same therapeutic technique results in such a variety of outcomes in different times, places, people, and settings.

The VA hospital, Ft. Harrison, Indianapolis, and Indiana were excellent settings at that time. The staff were intelligent and highly motivated. Innovations were tried after the approval by the chiefs of service, medicine, and professional service. Environments could be fairly well structured and results were evaluated carefully and objectively.

Building a Doctoral Program

After one year of college teaching and two-and-one-half years of professional experience, I joined the faculty of Florida State University at a time of growth and challenge. I plunged into the task of developing the Ph.D. program to gain APA (American Psychological Association) approval in clinical psychology. In addition to teaching four advanced graduate courses, directing thesis research, and the usual duties, I supervised and worked in a challenging mental health clinic, the Human Relations Institute of Leon County. This was an all-purpose clinic operated jointly, and usually cooperatively, by the County Health Department, the Department of Psychology and the School of Social Work of the university, the school system, plus some help from the community at large. Because it was a sort of confederation, it was not dominated by the medical model or the M.D.'s who *were* excellent professionals. The graduate students were mature (many were World War II veterans) and were able to explore many innovative approaches. We were also able to evaluate various therapeutic approaches and developed a degree of technical eclecticism which ranged from the unorthodox approach of Whitaker and Malone, to the most Rogerian, on to the most behavioral. Despite our diversity, or maybe because of it, we received APA approval of our Ph.D. clinical psychology program in 1954.

With time and experience, we moved further and further away from the approach of determining what is wrong and what can be done to fix it to the broader approach of looking at the total situation, the total person. We determined what the strengths and potential strengths were of the individual. Then we worked with him to determine goals and devised methods to achieve them, then reassessed the total situation to help him decide what the next phase should be. Because this was an active interaction between people, the client did not tend to become dependent as in psychoanalytic therapy nor stay in the phase of simply ventilating feelings without ever taking positive action, as was so often found in Rogerian therapy. Our ongoing program of critical self-evaluation revealed convincing evidence as to the effectiveness of different approaches with different types of clients. There were still events that simply supported the old saying, "Some people are helped by the darndest things."

Broadening the Field

Critical analyses led me to question the total contribution we were making to society. We had a good record of helping those who were marginal or inadequate to become more effective or adequate in their functioning. On the other hand, what were we doing with those who were already functioning adequately to all appearances, but had much unrealized potential? Would not society profit even more if these average or above average individuals led richer, more productive lives? Organizations for "exceptional children" had a stated purpose of studying and helping those who were exceptionally talented as well as those who were exceptional from the standpoint of impairment, yet practically all the effort went to the impaired—little or none to the talented. The significant percentage of dropouts who were of high potential was not attended to. While trying to do something about this, I encountered a group that was well ahead of me in this regard. The group was Rorher, Hibler, and Replogle, psychologists to management. Some of this group had been moving from evaluation, selection, and placement into the personal development of chief executive officers and other management and key personnel. This had an appeal. If an executive can be helped to become better adjusted, a better leader, a better developer of people, then many people benefit. Furthermore, here was a chance to learn what was not available on any campus, the study of the *interbehavior* of a variety of people in a variety of organizations working for a variety of purposes.

People in Organizations

In approximately five years of working with top management of research, service, educational, industrial, and even religious organizations, the place of interbehavioral psychology became more and more apparent. The methods and constructs of interbehaviorism were the only ones that came close to fitting the situations observed in such a setting. Many techniques—self-evaluation, tests, behavior observations, interviewing, and counseling—were applied, but integration and understanding needed a more comprehensive systems approach.

Another gratifying aspect of this work situation was further opportunity for evaluations of one's work. We constantly asked ourselves, "Are we doing any good?" There were many objective measures of organizational effectiveness. There were also chances for semicontrolled studies. For example, one would compare a division in which the psychological development programs were applied with those comparable divisions of the same corporation in which the program had not been applied.

As one would expect, the organization's development demands honesty, integrity, and self-discipline as well as ability. Steps of the program usually progress something like this: After one or more discussions with the chief executive on what can or cannot be done, a decision is made to go ahead. Some, as in a research institute in which I worked, involve sessions with the several division heads of the scientific disciplines represented in the institute. If the program is initiated, we work with the chief first, and only when we and the CEO together decide to do so is the program extended to the next level. Those professionals who have previous contacts with psychologists find this experience different, due to the comprehensive, positive, achievement-oriented approach and the process of interaction between people working together. This relationship is profoundly different from that of the "expert" telling someone what to do, or sitting passively and reflecting.

The consultant does not usurp management's functions nor tell the manager what to do. Questions, even unpleasant ones, are raised, attention is called to setting factors, and self-criticism is encouraged along with recognition of positive factors. While communication is facilitated, the psychologist does not become the communicator or the communication system. The psychologist does not work between people, but rather strengthens the relationship between and among people.

In addition to personal self-evaluation and development, the consulting psychologist works to help develop and repeatedly evaluate the organization as a whole, as an organism. Just as individuals look to their own strengths and weaknesses, opportunities and threats, the members of the organization do the same for the organization as a total system operating in the organization's milieu. Such a total system appeared in the space program.

Space Program

In the late 1950s some of our client organizations were engaged in the space program. Many of the issues which arose stimulated me to call on my background experience in human factors engineering at the Aviation Psychology Lab at Indiana University, the receptor processes and perception experiments under Hoisington (one of Titchener's outstanding products), and undergraduate engineering and physical science experience. In 1959 I joined the space medicine section of Indiana University to conduct applied research in manned space flight. In addition to laboratory and simulation research, I spent the next eleven years heading what was called "system effectiveness." This involved initiating and coordinating the system analysis, personnel subsystem, and human factors—reliability, maintainability, value engineering, and cost-effectiveness—integrating them with the hardware.

One of the most exciting benefits of the space program has been the merging of the psychological systems approach with the engineering systems approach. As was pointed out at a conference on interbehaviorism in Plattsburg, New York, in 1968, high-speed digital computers, systems-engineering developments, and manual and optimal control theory combined with interbehaviorism to give us a powerful tool for research and application.

As the system develops in concept and design, successive iterations involve change and expansion of more and more specific detail. Theoretical, computerized, and actual man-machine simulations add more and more realistic data and understanding to the complex interactions. The systems-oriented interbehaviorists participate from initial conceptual phases through final operation. Sometimes it takes about as long to select, train, and deploy the personnel as it does to build the hardware. Interestingly, in the early days of the U.S. manned space flight program, the engineering attitude was that man would be essentially a passive passenger—the system would be all automatic and controlled from the ground. As it turned out, six of the seven Project Mercury flights would have been failures had there not been a humann operator aboard to make decisions and to take over for various subsystem failures. These facts made an impact on the next space system, the two-man Gemini program. This was one of the most successful programs ever. The human was in the loop at almost all times.

Even after the Apollo disaster—a fire which resulted in the loss of three astronauts—in which many safety and human factors engineering requirements were violated, the system was corrected and the goals of the program were met. For a time, anyway, our approach was effectively utilized.

Although the space program was receiving less than 1 percent of federal expenditures and even though it paid off in thousands of ways, the political and media setting factors were such that manned space flight expenditures were drastically reduced. At this time we were trying to apply some of the space program–generated knowledge to complex problems such as improved education, poverty, employment of the hard-core unemployed, community-action programs, environmental issues, and other non-aerospace issues. We encountered some dramatic examples of Murphy's Law (If it is possible for things to go wrong, eventually they will) and Fuller's Law (If it is physically possible for things to go right, eventually they will). In short, you may not win them all, but you will not lose them all if you keep trying. The disappointments tended to be brought about by uncontrollable factors. In a program such as the Apollo moon exploration, everyone working in the program knew and approved of the goals of exploring the moon and returning safely; however, in our attempts to apply our approach to other problems, there was lacking anything resembling unanimity with respect to ultimate goals, much less the means to reach them.

One That Murphy Won

In the late 1960s and early 1970s our newly founded science systems organization set out to conquer some of the more pressing earthbound problems. One system was developed to make an impact on the hard-core unemployed. After a dramatic episode such as the riots in Watts or Detroit, a large number of persons from the area would be given jobs. A short time later, the majority would again be unemployed. Several factors were defined by our research. These included such factors as basic motivation and attitudes toward work and the work ethic in general. Many persons considered that the most "low-down, worthless" thing a person could do was to have a job and go to work daily. This had been stated to us many times. Another factor was the life-style and habits of the target population. Even when motivated to work, some people did not have the habit of being in any particular place at a particular time with regularity. (One employer-employee agreement was to involve the taxicab company; the taxicab dispatcher would call the employee in the morning, the cab driver would arrive at the appropriate time, and if the employee was not up and ready, the driver would enter the house and assure the employee's arrival at work on time.)

Once on the job, work needed to be accomplished with fellow workers and supervisors. Attitudes toward accepting instructions, parking in areas other than that of the chief executive and other reserved spaces, tolerance and productive interactions among the new and previously employed workers, and training in behaviors over and above the job skills as such were all part of our program development. The goal was not just to attain the placement of the difficult to employ, but to arrange an ongoing, iterative, comprehensive program that would assure continued successful employment for months and years to come. The unpredicted factor was finally teased out of the employment security personnel when they finally got through to us that their reinforcers—promotions, more money, more subordinates—were related to the number of people placed on a job rather than on successful or continuing job placements. Consequently, if a person was placed, quit or was fired, and placed again every month, twelve placements were credited. If a person was placed and stayed on the job the rest of the year, only one placement was credited. A similar experience was encountered in working with Aid to Dependent Children (ADC) recipients. After many clients left ADC following several short sessions with the psychologist, the program of offering psychological consultations paid for by Medicaid was discontinued. Oddly enough, a longer number of sessions and consequently less effective clinical services may have saved the problem.

You Cannot Lose Them All

There were also some successes. One program was conducted in a county in southern Michigan. Contacts were made initially with the administration of the education establishment. Eventually a meeting was held with the curriculum committee for the county educational system. Hours were spent in outlining the program and answering questions and objections posed by the forty persons involved at all levels of the K–12 school system. Some were skeptical at first because they were not sure the program would be effective; some were skeptical or reluctant because they feared the program would be too effective and it seemed dangerous to introduce anything that would be that effective; one woman had reservations due to the religious belief that "God has ordered that we punish wrong-doing." She recognized and accepted the proposition that more is accomplished through differential reinforcement whereby desired behavior is reinforced and the undesired behavior is weakened through extinction (ignoring it). The manner in which this objection was handled will remain forever a secret between God and us.

In addition to promulgating the plan, a graduate-level class was held for the participating teachers. Observer-coaches were provided for each class and the program director visited the classes periodically. The program of systematic, interbehavioral classroom management was tailored to fit each situation—the emotionally impaired, the intellectually impaired, the mainstream, the gifted. Statistically, the results were highly significant. The direct observations yielded a wealth of anecdotes and teaching aids which are still in use, more than a decade later. By all criteria the students learned more, behaved better, and improved adjustment, but the teachers, observer-coaches, and program manager all profited intellectually.

Back to the Classroom

The last two decades have afforded opportunities to apply the interbehavioral approach in the juvenile justice system and in institutions of higher learning such as Temple Buell (now a part of the University of Denver), University of Michigan—Grand Rapids Center, Aquinas College, and Muskegon Community College. Many students learn not only the academic materials but also the coping skills, more effective adjustment, and stress management following a broad systems approach.

Some college and university instruction is simply indoctrination. Some indoctrinate and train in a particular skill or set of skills (welding, computer programming); some try to educate in the traditional sense of the word. In many institutions today one encounters almost the complete range of human size, shape, intellectual level, and emotional adjustment. In the last ten years I have had in the same class people who have ''graduated'' from high school who fit and came through the programs for the intellectually impaired and people who were as brilliant as any Ph.D. candidate I ever met. Some read at the third-grade level and some read 600 words per minute with good comprehension and recall. Some have been psychotic, some have committed homicide. Some were prostitutes, some were virgins. When confronted with such classes, there are several alternatives. One alternative is to pass everyone. A second alternative is to set and maintain standards, present your materials in the classroom, make assignments, give tests, and eliminate those who do not perform. A more broad-based systems approach is to analyze the situation in light of the final goals one must be expected to reach and mutually build a program plan for each to reach the goal.

In addition to the academic learning goals for each course, every student has an opportunity, even as requirement, to perform some applied research. Many choose to work on themselves, their own behavior, or on that of someone in their immediate family or circle of intimates. The number of these projects now exceeds 5,000 and they are under continuous analysis for trends, relationships among the known factors, success indicators, new technique descriptions, and so on. Many are able to overcome problems which they have had for years, on which they have spent thousands of dollars for psychiatric and other therapies, and which they have found to be major obstacles in their careers and their lives. The gentleman who has given me permission to discuss his project was typical of those who solved a problem that thousands of dollars worth of traditional psychotherapy had yet to solve. The man in question was in his mid-thirties, married, a father of three. He was very sensitive to the subject of homosexuality. When the topic came into classroom or other discussions, he became agitated and left the room. He could not tolerate the presence of overt male homosexuals and had lost more than one good job on this account. His father had sexually molested him for some period in his youth and had verbally abused him in conjunction with the sexual abuse. He had such anger and hatred toward his father that he would drive out of his way in order to avoid his father's neighborhood for fear that if he saw him he might try to run him down with his automobile.

Early in the semester, the students were asked to work toward choosing a goal they wanted to accomplish without being too concerned with the means. In the case of this gentleman, the setting factors and the biographical history were determined. Then an inventory of all the various setting factors and their correlates was constructed. A program of self-analysis at a more extensive level was pursued at this point. Then a goal and a step-by-step program to reach that goal were set. Contingency plans came next with periodic updating and possible fine-tuning of the program. Various techniques were explored and tried. Realistic long-term goals were set and many short-term, partial landmark goals outlined. Analysis, self-instruction, support from peers, and a program of progressive desensitization followed. Midway in the semester, word came that the father had been seriously injured in an automobile collision. The son was practically forced by family pressure to visit the hospitalized father, so feared and hated. We went through some simulations or behavior rehearsals, some expressions of interpersonal support, and he was able to behave in a civilized fashion in the hospital—at first with the whole family there, later in a more private situation. Aside from the father-son interaction, he was able to desensitize himself completely and to behave in a neutral fashion around homosexuals and to handle the classroom discussions of the subject in a productive, nonthreatened manner.

Two years later, as many do, he returned to report on his life, on progress in general, and on his problem in particular. He expressed appreciation of what he had accomplished as part of his term project in class. He had recently come from his father's funeral. In the years following the automobile accident, he and his father had become fairly good friends. He had forgiven his father and developed some positive attitudes or feelings for him. His father too had changed through the understanding of his son. Some people feel guilt and remorse when someone, particularly a family member, dies and there is this history of anger, hatred, and even death wish. This former student recognized that and expressed gratitude for having been helped to cope with and overcome his problem so that he could feel at peace with his father before and after the father's death.

While many projects have been in the nature of the one just described, more are of a somewhat routine nature. People control their weight, toilet train their children, stop bad habits such as all sorts of substance abuse, telling lies, stopping at rest stops for casual sex, swearing, developing better study habits, and improving their sexual performance. People are not always entirely successful in reaching their goals in the alloted time. Some discover that they really did not want to do what they said they did in the first place. This is an achievement in itself. Many keep working.

Many students, particularly advanced undergraduate or graduate students, have been able to set up programs in their workplace. These have included the institution of numerical control (robotics) machinery and its integration with the people in the workplace; others have set up programs of substance-abuse treatment, safety, human factors engineering, personnel programs including productive affirmative-action programs, minority-owned and -operated business surveys and consulting, and programs for women in management. Meanwhile, they are learning objective, scientifically based principles of psychology, particularly interbehavioral psychology. Rather than a rat or dog lab or the traditional psychology laboratory, they find their laboratory is all around them; it is the field in which they live.

Summary

Many people have shared these last forty years in which attempts have been made to apply the data and methods of an objective, comprehensive, system-oriented interbehavioral psychology. While two books on bioastronautics and dozens of articles and technical reports (many of them published by the U.S. government) have come out of these efforts, the odyssey has not been publicized. I continue to teach and hope that I am getting the hang of it. I continue a broad spectrum of consultation with individuals and organizations. I have learned from many people and many situations and I am grateful to my mentors, particularly J. R. Kantor and B. F. Skinner. I also would like to thank the reader for staying with me this far—give yourself a reinforcer.

_____ *Part II*

Methods

4

The Interbehavioral Approach to Psychopathology

Robert W. Lundin

This chapter introduces the categorical scheme in J. R. Kantor's analysis of psychopathology first set down by him in 1926 (Kantor, 1926). Following a review of the various criteria of abnormality, concepts of personality will be discussed that reflect the basic principles of the interbehavioral position as they apply to the origin and development of pathological responding. Kantor's approach explains abnormal behavior as a function of the interbehavioral history and various setting factors as they operate in the life of an individual.

Since all human activity is a function of so many varied specific factors, differences in an individual's personality equipment are going to result—no two people have identical reactional biographies. Individual differences among people have been observed and recorded since earliest times. Some men were better farmers, while others were better hunters. Beginning in the latter part of the nineteenth century, Sir Francis Galton (1885) first applied Darwinian principles of variation to the human species. At the turn of the twentieth century A. Binet and T. Simon (1905) undertook the study of variation in intelligence, devising a technique for differentiating degrees of ability in school children.

The normal variations in behavior serve as the basis for our study of abnormal or pathological personalities. The interbehavioral approach has long abandoned terms such as "mental illness" or "mental disease" (McDougall, 1922). However, in psychiatric and other mentalistic circles the notation of the "sick mind" still abounds. The interbehavioral approach would rather speak of unusual, unadaptable, or pathological forms of interbehavior.

Individual differences in behavior derive from individual differences in both biological and psychological equipment. Kantor (1926) pointed out the role of defective biological equipment when he wrote of deteriorating and traumatic personalities as seen in the cases of senile and brain-injured persons.

Of even greater importance are individual differences in psychological equipment. Behavioral deficit, early impoverishment, and environmental deprivation all leave their marks on the personality of the individual. The sheltered or restricted child has been so protected that when actual contacts with outside stimuli arise, he or she is unequipped to respond appropriately, if at all.

In other cases the problem centers more closely around the development of inappropriate behavior. Unusual learning, perhaps as a result of an unconventional family upbringing, places unusual demands on a child, often at a time when he or she has to face other children. If he or she has developed contrary or peculiar patterns of behavior, the new demands may lead to maladaptive reactions.

Criteria of Abnormality

The criteria of behavior abnormalities depend upon the point of view one takes. If we were to suggest a *medical criterion* the emphasis would be on the individual's inability to carry out his or her biological processes. Gross deformities of the body or obstructions in glandular functioning are considered pathological. Although biological events may enter into our understanding of psychological abnormalities, they must not be accepted as the sole criterion by which we judge an individual's behavior.

On the other hand, the *legal criterion* encounters a different problem. The lawyer is faced with a person's responsibility for his or her acts. If a person's behavior involves liability for injuries to himself or herself or other people, that person will be considered pathological. Perhaps one's actions impinge upon those of a neighbor or result in destruction of that neighbor's property. From a legal standpoint a person may be judged sane or insane and treated accordingly. In the early and mid-nineteenth century little distinction was made between a severely disordered personality and an institutionalized criminal.

Somewhat related to the legal criterion is the *sociological criterion*. The sociologist is concerned with group conduct and the attitudes and beliefs of the community. The requirements of a group constitute the criterion for the judgment of abnormality.

Psychological Criteria

Interbehavioral history. In investigating the interbehavioral history of an individual we look into both the reactional biography and the stimulus evolution. As response functions are developed so also are stimulus functions acquired. Basically, the reactional biography refers to the history of interactions an individual has had with various stimulus objects. It is gradually built up from birth resulting in what Kantor calls an organism's *behavior equipment*. The stimulus evolution is the process of stimulus function development of objects in psycho-logical interbehavior. On the stimulus side it corresponds with the development of the reactional biography on the response side.

It is in the interbehavioral history that we find the origins of psychological difficulties. Here we will discover if a person's conduct is considered proper or not. As a result of inappropriate psychological development many failures of responding may occur. Likewise, as a result of an improper interbehavioral history, behavior will be deficient or maladaptive or, in some circumstances, disastrous.

Immediate behavior surroundings. Another view of abnormality is through inquiry into a person's immediate behavior surroundings still with reference to one's reactional biography. In the events of tremendous crisis such as floods, storms, or fire, the person is unprepared for adequate adaptation. Still these are extraordinary circumstances to which one must react. Through an inquiry of immediate behavioral surroundings we can appraise whether or not an individual, over the course of time, will be able to adjust to the trauma of the new situation. Thus, we conclude "that an adequate psychological criterion for pathological behavior conditions must be specific and particular—one which is derived from an intimate study of an individual and his reactional conditions and not from any type of statistical data concerning psychological conduct" (Kantor, 1926, p. 455).

Reaction system defects. Abnormal behavior characteristically arises out of some defect in the reaction system. Either the appropriate behavior has never been developed or for some reason it fails to function. First, the difficulty may be correlated with an anatomical structure or set of structures. Examples would include brain damage or improper development of the nervous system. Second, it may be that the person has never had the opportunity to acquire appropriate behavior equipment which would allow him or her to cope with the demands of a particular situation. Some forms of retardation would fit here. Bijou (1963) has suggested several possibilities: (1) children reared in isolated communities with minimum economic means, (2) children reared in institutions in which most social and emotional contacts usually found in a family are absent, and (3) children in families whose parents are emotionally disturbed and who prevent their offsprings from having usual interactions with people and other objects.

Third, we have the possibility of the acquisition of unsuitable reaction systems. Here we have individuals who have developed inappropriate reaction equipment so they are not able to react at all.

Finally, we have behavior segment difficulties where intended reactions with objects take on unusual or unsatisfactory stimulus functions. Extreme anxiety reactions, phobias, and compulsions to touch everything are all examples.

There are also cases where normally developed reactions to stimuli fail to operate when the stimulus object is present. The objects fail to perform their stimulus functions even though the appropriate reactions actually do exist for them. Typical examples are what the American Psychiatric Association (1980) now calls dissociative and conversion reactions. These include functional paralyses, anesthesias, mutism, anorexia, and amnesias.

On the basis of the principles of classification of behavioral abnormality, Kantor (1926) places the difficulties into three main divisions with a number of subdivisions under each. The reason for the divisions is to point out the various ways in which behavioral abnormalities develop and operate. In investigating abnormal behavior we always begin with a particular individual and the characteristics of his or her conduct. Kantor (1926) has identified the three main divisions as (1) unusual behavior, (2) unadaptive behavior, and (3) defective or pathological behavior. These same terms also refer to the personalities performing the behavior.

Unusual Personalities

The unusual personality is not ordinarily listed in the traditional classification systems; for example, the recent classification system of the American Psychiatric Association (1980) DSM (Diagnostic and Statistical Manual) III, perhaps because these are borderline cases (Lundin, 1965). Yet, a description of unusual personalities is legitimately a part of abnormal psychology, so the unusual personality forms a link in the continuum from more conventional modes of conduct considered normal to the most pathological.

That group of individuals described as unusual has developed some extreme variation of normal behavior patterns, but these patterns are not unadaptable. For example, we may note the eccentric who is noticed for his or her idiosyncrasies but gets along perfectly well in managing his or her affairs and in taking care of him- or herself. These unusual behavior patterns need not interfere with the ordinary adjustments that individuals make to their material and social surroundings. Their behavior may be quite exaggerated and they distinguish themselves for their peculiarities.

In some cases only a few behavior patterns are unusual. Here we could include a person who had some peculiar mannerism such as an unusual way of speaking or a peculiar set of attitudes, perhaps with regard to matters of religion or politics. These behaviors distinguish the individual markedly from other members of the group.

Then there are cases of individuals with many behavior patterns considered unusual. A typical example might be foreigners who come into a particular group in which there is a different language and set of customs and manners. On the other hand, there are individuals with a limited number of eccentricities, but these eccentricities are so overshadowing that the rest of the personality appears distinctly different from the rest of mankind. In this group we might include the temperamental orchestra conductor or opera singer who is able to get by because of extreme talent and the behavior of others may be directed to his or her own whims of the moment. Other possibilities include the dreamer who spends his or her time building castles in the air, the person who talks of great ideas but accomplishes nothing. At the other extreme is the person who is constantly trying new things with only an occasional success.

Kantor (1926) suggests that cases of genius should be included in this group of unusual personalities. These are individuals who because of some great talent or ability have set themselves aside from others and who have left behind great accomplishments of artistic, musical, or scientific creation.

Unadaptable Personalities

Unadaptable personalities are those who are unable to adapt themselves to their social or natural surroundings. The behavior of these individuals either prevents them from getting along with other people or interferes with their general welfare. Their behavior or lack of it may make them undesirable neighbors or prevent them from earning a living or lead to unsatisfactory living conditions.

Kantor (1926) suggests that the simplest cases of unadaptable behavior are the shy, bashful, or retiring persons who cannot meet people on equal terms or face their surroundings. In this group we also place the "snoops" and "busybodies" who interfere with the privacies and intimacies of others. Likewise included is the persistent salesman whose unreserved insistence has complete disregard for a prospect's convenience and dignity.

Also included among the unadaptable personalities are chronic gripers, those individuals who persistently criticize and disapprove of their surrounding conditions and people about them. They condemn the activities of others on religious, moral, and political issues. Often these people are new to a community. Accordingly, they belittle their new surroundings and protest against them in favor of their previous environment. These are the "free thinkers" who find it difficult or impossible to abide by the conventional and moral standards of a given society. Here we also include conscientious objectors who because of various previously acquired principles cannot participate in war activities of the group and as a result find their attitudes deviant from the consensus.

Criminal Personalities

From a psychological point of view the criminal personality has developed behavior equipment whereby he or she reacts without regard for the rights or privileges of others. Criminal behavior equipment may be acquired because of the sheer necessity of one's living conditions. In other instances it may be necessary to defend oneself against other persons or groups that are hostile. This group would include juvenile gangs that compete for territories and goods. In these cases there are individuals whose antisocial conduct has been acquired in contact with and entirely approved by a particular group which in turn causes inconvenience and harm to the public at large.

Anxious Personalities

Perhaps Freud (1936) was the first to recognize the significance of anxiety in the development of maladaptive behavior. Cases of chronic and acute anxiety interfere with the normal course of living. Anxious individuals appear to be miserable and unhappy. The normal transitory fears that are part of everyday living become prolonged. There are difficulties in sleep, loss of appetite, stiffness of the muscles, and failure of concentration and memorial reactions. From time to time anxiety attacks may occur. These are episodes of behavioral disorganization in which an already anxious behavior becomes intensified. Often the person cannot identify the stimulus conditions that precipitate these reactions. At other times the attacks may be set off by apparently insignificant stimuli such as a mere disappointment, the loss of an order in business, a poor mark in school, or the cancellation of a social engagement. The person quite suddenly becomes restless and can no longer continue at what he or she is doing. There may be a shivering sensation or a feeling of panic. The disorganization may become quite intense leaving the individual unable to decide where to go or what to do. This is an exaggeration of normal fear.

Defective or Pathological Personalities

In this last and by far the largest division are the cases of persons whose behavior is decidedly irregular and unfit. Here we find the failure of particular reactions to operate when they are required, either because of inhibitions or because they are not part of a person's behavior equipment. An example of the first condition might be a person who has previously learned to speak but on a particular occasion is rendered mute or whose verbal responses are unintelligible. In the second condition we might find an individual who has never acquired a necessary mode of behavior.

Kantor (1926) has subdivided these pathological or defective personalities into various groups according to certain outstanding features of their behavior equipment. These include sources or types of origin of the abnormality, the limitations of the behavior, the specific kind of action that is pathological, and the effects of the abnormal conduct. These divisions are intended only for pragmatic purposes of orientation with regard to understanding any particular kind of psychological disorder. Kantor (1926) made clear that he was not intending to pigeonhole abnormal individuals into separate categories, allowing that any single individual's total behavioral abnormalities might place him or her into several classifications. However, for purposes of discussion, he identifies the various groups or personalities into the following: (1) undeveloped, (2) defectively developed, (3) disintegrated, (4) dissociated, (5) degenerating, (6) disorganized, and (7) traumatic.

Undeveloped Personalities

Undeveloped personalities are individuals with various degrees of retardation. On the basis of the degree of retardation, the American Association for Mental Deficiency (1977) has classified the individuals based on the Binet IQ into mildly retarded, moderately retarded, severly retarded, and profoundly retarded. In older psychological classifications these individuals were called "feebleminded." From the point of view of origin of the abnormality these persons have been unable to acquire the appropriate reaction systems which would allow them to function appropriately in a normal society, either because they have never had contact with the necessary stimulus objects (environmental deficiency) or because of an inability to acquire reaction systems even where the contact with the objects was possible. In these latter cases the development of appropriate behavior is impossible because it is correlated with certain biological limitations or defects.

In the instances of environmental deficiency, Kantor (1926) cites the "Strange Case of Kasper Hauser" described by Tredgold (1922). Cases of nondevelopment correlated with biological defects include brain injury, microcephaly, cretinism, hydrocephaly, Down's syndrome, or conditions correlated with infectious disease such as syphilis, encephalitis, or meningitis.

In other cases of behavior segment defects there are individuals who so devote themselves to one occupation that the rest of their personality equipment is lacking. Here we find artists or scientists who are incapable of responding to their economic or social surroundings.

Kantor liked to point out to his classes that we are all "feebleminded" to the degree that some of us might never have developed reaction systems which allow us to interact with musical, artistic, mechanical, or athletic stimulus objects.

With regard to the hereditary factors operating in the nondevelopment of certain personalities, Kantor (1926) stedfastly maintained that only to the degree that these are related to structural impediments can they be allowed as explanations. In other words, heredity does not operate in environmental deficiencies.

Defective Personalities

The principal behavioral characteristic of individuals with defective personalities is the development of wrong behavior equipment so that they are unable to adjust themselves to their natural and social surroundings. Here the emphasis is on undesirable or maladjusted behavior. This maladjustment leaves the person unfit to react appropriately to certain situations.

Delinquent personalities. Kantor (1926) cites delinquent personalities as the first example of defective behavior organization. These people do not adjust to the legal and social norms or moral institutions which constitute part of their cultural surroundings. Here we would find individuals with sexual deviations: homosexuals, transvestites, people with particular fetishes, sadists, masochists, and pedophiliacs.

Likewise, in this group would be sociopaths or what DSM III (1980) identifies as antisocial personalities. These persons cannot function adequately in their social surroundings. Their pathological lying, cheating, and swindling chronically get them in trouble and they seldom operate to their own advantage. As Cleckley (1955) has pointed out, they seem to go out of their way to make a failure of life.

Paranoid personalities. People with paranoid personalities exhibit abnormalities in their thinking behavior. They make false inferences with regard to their observations of their surroundings. DSM III (1980) identifies these individuals as being suspicious, hypersensitive, rigid, envious, and argumentative. Instead of recognizing their own faults and failures, they will ascribe their wrong behavior to others. They accuse others of trickery and look for evidence to substantiate their false beliefs.

In more extreme cases designated as paranoia, the behavior becomes delusional. These individuals believe that they are singled out, taken advantage of, plotted against, stolen from, spied upon, or mistreated by their enemies. The delusions usually center on a particular theme: a job, an invention, or financial matters. Although the evidence may be overwhelmingly contrary to their claims, they are unwilling to accept any plausible explanation.

Although delusions of persecution tend to dominate their behavior, many paranoid individuals express delusions of grandeur. They may believe they have unique or special talents or have created remarkable inventions or made unique discoveries. Frequently, their delusional reactions can be particularly convincing to those unaware of the actual facts.

The seriousness of the paranoid behavior depends on the number of forms it takes as well as the importance of the situation and the length of time it has been developing.

Catatonic personalities. Individuals with catatonic personalities have developed feeling responses that are negativistic in nature. They become progressively disinterested in their surroundings. They become apathetic and if the behavior loss progresses far enough, they appear to be comatose or stuporous. Their regressive behavior may continue to the point where they fail to take care of their elementary biological functions. They lack concern for the conventions of social life or with adapting themselves to their surroundings.

Schizophrenic personalities. Kantor describes schizophrenic personalities as exhibiting a progressive detachment from the environing world of work and responsibility (1926). Previously in excellent contact with their social institutions and economic surroundings, they begin to fall away from these attachments. This withdrawal from their usual activities and responsibilities presents a marked contrast to their previous behavioral interactions. An active businessman becomes listless and indifferent to his work, finally losing contact with his former surroundings. In some cases all that remains is the performance of certain mannerisms or gestures bearing some possible relationship to his former work. Kantor (1926) attributes the schizophrenic personality to long drawn out difficulties in the development of a person's reactional biography. Early in life these individuals encounter certain difficulties with which they cannot cope. In the early stages they appear shy and timid and do not participate in the same activities as others of their own age. Later on they substitute their own imaginative reactions to replace situations which actually surround them in the natural world. More specifically, Kantor (1926) cites economic and social difficulties with which the person cannot adjust. An inability to compete with others in various endeavors—economic, intellectual, social, or artistic—leads these people to give up. Instead, they develop behavior equipment that is of no use in these critical situations. At the basis of the development of the schizophrenic abnormality may exist "a general functional inferiority of the biological individual" (Kantor, 1926, p. 484). Such a functional abnormality may result in an inferior person or it may lead the individual to develop withdrawing and detached behavior.

Hypochondriacal personalities. The pathological behavior equipment of hypochondriacal individuals centers around health stimulus situations in some way or form. Because of certain circumstances to be found in their behavioral surroundings, they develop responses of fatigue, over concern for disease and health or mistaken attitudes regarding their own bodily functioning. In many cases these concerns and misbeliefs result in an inability to cope with the demands of everyday living. The most extreme forms include the psychological invalids who take to their beds with numerous imagined physical complaints as a protection against the external demands placed on them. In many cases these persons demand much care and attention. (Freud called this the secondary gain in the neurosis.) They demand to be pampered and protected from disease conditions. In their developmental histories, they have learned to be fearful and anxious of germs. Over time they build up more and more invalid-type reactions. As with other kinds of pathological responding, certain specific conditions favor the development of this particular condition. Some could relate to visual or hearing difficulties, an early prolonged illness, being frail as a child, or oversolicitous parents even in cases of minor illness.

Compulsive personalities. Kantor (1926) describes compulsive individuals as having no control over their own actions, behaving without premeditation or foresight with results that appear to be either unsatisfactory or even disastrous. In the presence of a particular stimulus or set of stimuli their reactions appear completely automatic. Compulsive behavior may not only be quite inappropriate to the immediate circumstances but often in direct conflict with the rest of a person's organized behavior. Kantor (1926) has stressed the fact that these reactions are often merely exaggerations of what appear to be normal acts. Some examples include compulsive eating, drinking, handwashing, toothbrushing, or orderliness. In other cases we find the compulsive behavior to be a violation of the social norms. Cases of compulsive stealing, fire setting, or some aberrant sexual acts would fit here.

Compulsive behavior may have its origin in the play activities of children as well as the many rituals of parliamentary procedures, church liturgies, or fraternal rites. Children's games are often orderly and repetitious. We may observe little girls playing hopscotch or a small boy walking down a sidewalk saying, "Step on a crack, break your mother's back," as he goes out of his way to avoid any crack or break in the pavement. Preschool children and kindergarteners alike love to hear the same story read over and over again. In adult society, legal documents and proceedings are often compulsively arduous. Rules of etiquette and good form often seem arbitrary or even foolish to those unacquainted with them.

Closely correlated with compulsive personalities are the inhibitive and vacillating individuals. Here we may find an individual who hesitates lengthily before performing a certain act. He or she may consider it in all details, questioning the necessity for doing or not doing it or speculating about all of its consequences. Even after considering all possible ramifications he or she may do what was originally intended by the stimulus situation or after so much deliberation may not act at all.

Ordinarily, we may trace the beginnings of this vacillating or inhibitive behavior to certain prior conditions in the person's interbehavioral history. Perhaps as a child this person was constantly admonished and criticized. In other cases, the origin may have been a disaster which occurred just before or after an act had been performed.

Disintegrating Personalities

The characteristics of disintegrating personalities involve behavior that has been quite stable and normal up to a certain point following which there is a quite rapid loss of integrated activity. The disturbance involves a breaking down of previously organized behavior. In extreme cases, such as an acute manic attack or grand mal epileptic seizure, there is a complete explosion of the personality organization. One's reaction equipment may become violently disruptive. The degree of disruption differs from one case to another so the criterion of behavior exaggeration fits these cases very well. Some epileptic seizures are very slight amounting to little more than an "absence" in responding while others might be so violent that an onlooker might wonder how the person will survive the seizure. The same holds for attacks of manic excitement which can vary from slightly euphoric behavior in which there is little behavior disintegration to a hyperacute manic attack involving severe emotional explosions.

The principle of personality disintegration can be applied to other kinds of behavior disorder as well. These may include simple fainting, the temper tantrums of a child, or debilitating migraine headaches in adults.

Manic and depressive reactions. According to Zilboorg (1941) manic and depressive reactions have been known since ancient times. Hippocrates in the fourth century B.C. wrote of mania and melancholia.

Kantor (1926), along with many other psychologists (Cameron & Magaret, 1951; Cameron, 1963; Lundin, 1965), has pointed out that manic and depressive episodes occur when an individual is faced with the necessity for action in a situation that he or she cannot effectively meet. Extremely overwhelming conditions may lead directly to behavior disintegration: a death in the family, financial or social loss, destruction of property, or sudden disillusionment. Kantor (1926) also points out that striking changes in a person's general biological functioning and health may precipitate manic or depressive reaction patterns. Such conditions as childbirth, sexual maturation, or menopause may also precipitate an attack.

Cameron (1947) has likened the mild manic attack to mild alcoholic intoxication. The person is jolly, witty, expressing a high degree of self-confidence and rapid speech. In more severe cases the behavior is overactive with a rapid and intense verbal output. The person jumps from one topic of conversation to another. Frequently, overaggressive or hostile behavior is present.

Depressive episodes are characterized by feelings of sadness and melancholia. There is a slowing down of activity and speech. Kantor (1926) notes that the depressive personality often reverts to more infantile modes of reaction. Arieti (1959) reports that ideational reactions of suicide occur in 75 percent of cases and actual suicidal attempts in 10 to 15 percent of cases.

Dissociated Personalities

In dissociated personalities we are dealing with individuals whose behavior patterns have been either disrupted or disjointed, but often in a very orderly way. In one group now designated by DSM III (1980) as conversion reactions, there is a failure of proper behavior function (Kantor, 1926, refers to these as hysterical personalities). In a second group, reactive dissociation, there is an actual cleavage or splitting of some behavior from the rest of the personality organization. In either type, the difficulty goes back to the earlier developmental process. Responses have evolved that simply do not hang together very well. An individual grows up in an environment in which various objects and persons do not constitute a homogeneous unity. Later, under conditions of stress or frustration, the various parts of the behavior equipment separate along definite lines of cleavage and in their expression constitute various alterations and dissociations of the personality. The most extreme cases are represented in the multiple personality as described by Prince (1908) in the case of Miss Beauchamp and Thigpen and Cleckley (1957) in the *Three Faces of Eve*.

Conversion reactions. Kantor (1926) originally referred to cases of conversion reaction as "hysterical." Here certain reaction systems are held in abeyance or do not function when the appropriate stimulus objects are present. In these instances the dissociation takes the form of a nonfunctioning part of the behavior equipment. Ordinarily, in these instances there may be only a specific reaction system out of function. Thus, a person is unable to perform a certain type of action as if that person had never acquired the reaction system. Here are included the great varieties of amnesia. These losses of memorial behavior may only pertain to certain people or events and are limited to a given period of time. In other cases, the individual's loss is more general when he or she is unable to remember his or her own name or anything in his or her entire past history. Other kinds of conversion reactions may involve the loss of sensory functions as in cases of hysterical blindness, deafness, anesthesias, motor losses in paralyses, or linguistic failures in functioning. Grinker and Spiegel (1945) cite cases of rapid loss of sensory functions incurred under conditions of combat during World War II. Once the stress of combat was over, the lost function returned. It should be remembered that in all cases of functional loss the organs and nervous system were in no way damaged or diseased.

Alternating or multiple personalities. In cases of alternating or multiple personalities, the people do not lose part of their behavior equipment but use their equipment in alternating periods. The line of division between the personalities and the ways in which the alternations will occur depends on the original development of the personality. It must be realized that during the course of an individual's development the various reaction systems which constitute the entire personality were developing under entirely different auspices, so they were not subject to the same behavioral processes that ordinarily characterize the normal personality. We must look for the situation responsible for the alternation and check out the specific circumstances which precipitated the dissociation.

In a sense, we are all multiple personalities. As William James (1890) suggested many years ago, a person has as many different social selves as there are distinct groups or persons for whose opinion that person cares. A man might have different organizations of behavior for his minister, his mother or father, his fiancée, or the boys in his poker club. As normal individuals we are able to resolve these differences or allow them to operate specifically for different situations.

Degenerating Personalities

In this group of pathological personalities we find all those individuals who show a progressive degeneration of behavior. Ordinarily, these persons have developed normally without any undesirable or defective behavior equipment. At some particular point in their lives they begin to show a more or less rapid degeneration in their actions in the sense that they lose permanently certain aspects of previously acquired behavior. In some cases the decline may be very rapid. In others, the degeneration may occur slowly over a period of years.

In degenerating personalities, ordinarily, there are biological factors participating in the behavior decline such as infectious disease of the nervous system or cerebral degeneration accompanying aging.

Senile personalities. In this group are found cases of cerebral arteriosclerosis, senile dementia, and Alzheimer's disease. Of particular significance is the deterioration of memorial behavior, particularly for recent events. These people may readily recall events that occurred thirty years ago but cannot remember what they did yesterday. Furthermore, they have trouble integrating new behavior into previously established behavior patterns. Along with a decline in memorial responding is a decline in the maintenance of earlier established levels of activity. Previously acquired skills in mathematics, verbal reasoning, and linguistic communication decline. The businessperson may become negligent and inefficient in managing his affairs. A homemaker becomes sloppy and careless about caring for the home. Both may be careless about maintaining their personal appearance and matters of cleanliness and hygiene. In the final stages, the person becomes utterly confused and disoriented in time and space and cannot identify familiar people or places.

Paretic personalities. Paretic personalities have a condition in which an infectious disease is involved. The syphilis spirochaete has invaded the brain. In this instance the degeneration is more rapid than in the cases of senile degeneration. There are difficulties in speech and locomotion involving the loss of reflexes. There are also memory losses, confusion, and disorientation. The degeneration may also involve delusions and hallucinations.

Disorganized Personalities

Kantor (1926) describes disorganized personalities as inaccurate in their failure to connect properly with stimuli. Disorganized behavior is not the result of improper behavior development or acquisition. The difficulties are to be found in conditions that incoordinate the behavior or result in a loss of action.

The conditions of disorganization most commonly result from ingestion of a variety of drugs: alcohol, marijuana, cocaine, barbiturates, or opium. Other substances leading to disorganization would include a variety of poisons such as lead or gas. Infections resulting in high fever are also included as participants in disorganized behavior. In acute cases of intoxication with drugs, the behavior can be described as delirious. This involves an incapability of performing any organized perceptual or ideational conduct concerning other persons and things in their surroundings. The disorganization may apply to intellectual as well as moral behavior.

Another kind of disorganized behavior not involving drugs, poisons, or infections would result from excessive stress situations. In DSM III (1980) these conditions are described as "posttraumatic stress reactions." Here the precipitating factors could be misfortunes of all sorts: a business failure, loss of a family member, realization of infidelity of a spouse, or more individual catastrophes such as the destruction of one's home by fire or flood, extreme poverty, or economic disaster such as occurred during the Great Depression.

Traumatic Personalities

The normal individual is considered to be a biological unit. In the traumatic personality, behavior is broken up or destroyed because of organic destruction or the loss of an organ or part of an organ. In considering a person as a biological unit as well as a total behaving personality, we find when an organ is lost or put out of function the person is unable to perform activities that involve the use or operation of the lost or impaired organ. These biological losses will vary in degree and kind and differ according to the specific character of the injury. People so impaired are called traumatic.

Kantor (1926) distinguishes between two types of traumas, the generalized and the specialized. Under the generalized, he places those personalities where a defect, injury, or destruction is strategic to a whole class of behavior and where a variety of adjustments to behavioral situations might be involved. We would include here brain injuries or damage to other parts of the nervous system which would interfere with the performance of many activities. Brain tumors or gunshot wounds to the head would also be examples.

Under the more specialized traumas we would include behavioral deficits which are a function of more particular organs and where the defects are more localized. These would include loss or destruction of the eyes, ears, limbs, or hands resulting in the loss of eyesight, deafness, or the ability to walk or hold or throw things. Such injuries could involve organ deformities which lead to the insufficient functioning of glands such as sex, thyroid, or pituitary.

The Usefulness of Classification Systems

The discussion of traumatic personalities concludes Kantor's analysis of the kinds of pathological personalities. These descriptions are not all-inclusive but are intended as examples of one kind of classification system. Any schemes of classification are useful only if they aid in the understanding of any particular personality and its surroundings. A classification system is useless if it does not throw light upon our understanding of pathological personalities.

In conclusion, Kantor (1926) states that his system of classification and descriptions can serve only as reference points in a consideration of abnormal behavior. In comparison to other systems, in particular DSM III (1980), Kantor's system has certain advantages. First of all, it is not based on the medical model which considers behavior disorders as "mental diseases." This implies a psychophysical parallelism with "physical diseases." Second, it is based on a valid psychological principle, that of individual differences which applies to all forms of human responding. We start with unusual personalities, who express the mildest or least deviant characteristics. We then continue on to the more disruptive or unadaptable personalities and end with the most defective or pathological personalities. Third, the system is based on a description of different behavior characteristics which can be applied to separate classes of personality disorders. For example, the undeveloped personalities refer to nondevelopment or a lack of behavior acquisition, whereas disintegrated personalities involve normal behavior that is followed by a quite rapid and sudden loss of integrated activity. Likewise, dissociated personalities show a cleavage or splitting of some behavior from the rest of the personality organization. Finally, the system is based not on specific symptomatology as found in a medical handbook but on reliable behavioral descriptions of how people act differently as a result of their different interbehavioral histories. It is hoped that an understanding of the development of this approach to the study of psychopathology should aid in the various treatment approaches that follow in this book.

References

American Association for Mental Deficiency. 1977. *Manual on terminology and classification in mental retardation*. Washington, D.C.: AAMD.

American Psychiatric Association. 1980. *Diagnostic and statistical manual of mental disorders*, 3rd ed. Washington, D.C.: APA

Arieti, S. 1959. *American handbook of psychiatry*. New York: Basic Books.

Bijou, S. W. 1963. Theory and research in mental (developmental) retardation. *Psychological Record* 13: 95–116

Binet, A., and T. Simon. 1905. Methodes novelles pour la diagnostic intellectual des anormaux. *Année Psychologie* II: 191–224.

Cameron, N. 1947. *The psychology of behavior disorders*. Boston: Houghton Mifflin.

Cameron, N. 1963. *Personality development and psychopathology: A dynamic approach*. Boston: Houghton Mifflin.

Cameron, N., and A. Magaret, 1951. *Behavior pathology*. Boston: Houghton Mifflin.

Cleckley, H. 1955. *The mask of sanity*, 3rd ed. St. Louis: Mosby.

Freud, S. 1936. *Inhibitions, symptoms and anxiety*. London: Hogarth Press.

Galton, F. 1885. *Inquiries into the human faculty and its development*. London: Macmillan.

Grinker, R. R., and J. P. Spiegel. 1945. *Man under stress*. New York: Blakiston.

James, W. 1890. *Principles of psychology*. New York: Holt.

Kantor, J. R. 1926. *Principles of psychology*, vol. II. New York: Alfred A. Knopf.

Lundin, R. W. 1965. *Principles of psychopathology*. Columbus, Ohio: Merrill.

McDougall, W. 1922. The nature of mental diseases. *American Journal of Psychiatry* 78:335–55.

Prince, M. 1908. *The dissociation of a personality*. New York: Longman, Green.

Thigpen, C. H., and H. Cleckley. 1957. *The three faces of Eve*. New York: McGraw-Hill.

Tredgold, A. F. 1922. *Mental deficiency*. New York: William Woods.

Zilboorg, G. 1941. *A history of medical psychology*. New York: Norton.

5

An Interbehavioral Approach to Clinical Child Psychology: Toward an Understanding of Troubled Families

Robert G. Wahler and Della M. Hann

In the past twenty years applied behavior analysis (ABA) has forged a place of its own among the strategic approaches in psychology. Since the early years of ABA utilization, the strategy has gained popularity in guiding research and applied work on a wide range of human problems. Not unexpectedly, the guiding principles encompassed within ABA have expanded from the early focus on relatively simple problems to the more complex behavior ecology issues defining today's problem topics (see Rogers-Warren & Warren, 1977). While this expansion is evident in a number of specialty fields of psychology, the clinical child specialty is one of the most active in this respect. Assessment and treatment operations with troubled children, their parents, siblings, teachers, and peers continue to be guided by the basic and well-known three-term operant principle (discriminative stimulus, response, reinforcement). However, it is also evident that clinical investigators are considering stimulus and response functions more complex than those summarized in the familiar operant concept. On the stimulus side, environmental *context* has been viewed as influencing operant processes in a manner not yet clearly understood. For example, K. D. O'Leary and R. E. Emery (1984) concluded that discordant marital relationships are associated with child behavior problems, while Wahler and Dumas (1985) reached a similar conclusion concerning the stimulus influence of socioeconomic disadvantage and parental conflict with extrafamily members of a community. In both surveys of the empirical literature, the marital, socioeconomic, and extrafamilial stressors were described as contextual stimuli for the troublesome parent-child relationships. In other words, the investigators were inclined to view parent-child reinforcement exchanges as indirectly determined by a third source of stimuli.

Neither set of investigators could document explanatory factors in the "indirect" stimulus-control process.

With respect to new looks at response functions, *response covariation* has become a phenomenon of interest for both researchers and practitioners. There are ample data to show that some responses in a child's repertoire are interdependent in the sense that rate changes in one are followed by predictable rate changes in others (see Kazdin's review, 1982). For example, Wahler and Fox (1980) found that the solitary toy play of three conduct-disordered children was inversely correlated with their day-to-day rule-violating behaviors. Then, when planned increases were produced in the children's solitary play, expected decreases were observed in their rule violations. The interesting conceptual feature of such response "clusters" or "classes" concerns their yet unknown organizational properties. While the covariations could be due to sequential stimulus-response chains (e.g., Strain & Ezzell, 1978), mediating autonomic respondent processes (Rescorla & Solomon, 1967), or some common reinforcer (Skinner, 1953), none of these possibilities have much empirical backing (see Voeltz & Evans, 1982). As in the case for stimulus context, the response covariation phenomenon remains as a puzzling but potentially useful descriptive concept.

These conceptual expansions within ABA, emerging only within recent years, reflect a conservative stance not shared by the more basic research cousins of ABA—proponents of the experimental analysis of behavior (TEAB). TEAB researchers such as C. Ferster and O. Lindsley (see Ullmann & Krasner, 1965) actually set the stage for the ABA movement through their laboratory demonstrations of operant processes in child behavior. Since these early demonstrations, TEAB investigators have continued their basic research studies, and their collective focus on behavioral processes has stepped beyond the three-term operant principle. For example, laboratory studies of "behavioral contrast" (Reynolds, 1961), "response independent reinforcement" (Sizemore & Lattal, 1977), "establishing operations" (Michael, 1982), and "behavioral hierarchies" (Bernstein & Ebbsen, 1976) refer to phenomena that are difficult to comprehend if one expects an explanation in terms of temporally immediate stimulus contingencies. As E. K. Morris, S. T. Higgens, and W. K. Bickel (1982a) point out, TEAB investigators have often resorted to descriptive concepts in their searches for understanding. In particular, the notion that responses occur in *units* specific to the individual organism has far-reaching implications. For some individuals, under some circumstances, a response might amount to relatively discrete actions (e.g., a lever press). Under other conditions, the response unit could be considerably broader in time and behavioral output (e.g., a thirty-minute sequence of walking, talking, and work). Since the defining property of the unit is its stimulus contingencies, there is no reason to believe that one could "catalog" an individual's response units with the expectation that this person would always behave according to the unit definition. As the environmental contingencies change, so will the response unit change. Thus, if we are perplexed in witnessing an animal's prolonged lever pressing with an electric shock consequence, a more *molar* assessment of the animal's behavior might prove instructive. As TEAB researchers have shown, such an organism will respond in that manner if some larger unit of its behavior is shaped under stimulus contingencies (Herrnstein & Hineline, 1966; Lambert, Bersh, Hineline, & Smith, 1973). In this case, our perplexity was due to witnessing a molecular component of some larger response unit.

Just as TEAB researchers have demonstrated how individuals can vary in response structure, similar analyses have shed light on *stimulus* units. Once again, the breadth of an environmental event that functions as a stimulus for an organism can be shown to depend on that organism's history of behavior-environment experiences. A discrete event, such as social approval, can function as a stimulus, but a *relationship* between or among events can also serve exactly the same function. Thus, in studies of multiple and concurrent reinforcement schedules, it is possible to generate stimulus control in which events independent of some targeted response serve to control that response (McKearney & Barrett, 1975). Perhaps the best-known example of this phenomenon is seen in laboratory demonstrations of behavioral contrast. G. S. Reynolds (1961), working with pigeons, established concurrent reinforcement schedules in which two stimuli served as discriminative events for the two schedules. Despite the independence of these schedules, planned changes in one schedule were shown to affect the animals' response rates when the second schedule was signaled. Even though the two discriminative stimuli signaled separate and independent reinforcement for responding, the animals behaved as if the stimuli were components of a single stimulus class.

Unusual stimulus-class phenomena, such as behavioral contrast, have also been shown to occur with humans. Thus, S. J. Simon, T. Ayllon, and M. A. Milan (1982) showed that children in school classroom settings are subject to the contrast form of stimulus control. When a sample of children who worked in two independent classroom settings received token reinforcement for academic performance, a withdrawal of reinforcement in one setting had predictable effects on the children's performance in the second setting. That is, academic response rate dropped in the classroom under extinction conditions and increased in the second classroom even though the reinforcement schedule in this classroom was unchanged. In another stimulus-class demonstration, S. A. Fowler and D. M. Baer (1981) were able to generate control over the sharing behavior of preschoolers through the use of noncontingent reinforcers. This sort of "superstitious" stimulus control (see Herrnstein, 1961) was established in a free-play setting by instructional and reinforcement operations conducted in an earlier free-play setting. The children were first instructed to share in the earlier setting and were reinforced by tokens for that behavior. Then, when token deliveries for early setting sharing were merely *delayed* until the day's end, the children also increased their sharing rates in the later setting—even though they were never reinforced for that behavior. Although token deliveries were only randomly connected to sharing in this second setting, the children behaved *as if* the deliveries were contingent. Much the same as in the behavioral-contrast studies, stimuli independent of a targeted response exercised control over that behavior.

Just as behavioral researchers have puzzled over the response covariation phenomenon, the above stimulus-class demonstrations are difficult to explain in terms of discrete and contingent stimuli. Stimulus units, like response units, appear to vary according to the individual's historical experiences. For some individuals, under some circumstances, a stimulus might amount to a relatively discrete event (e.g., social approval). Under other conditions, the unit could constitute a relationship among multiple events, none of which bear a contingent relationship to the behavior under control. As we shall see, the clinical implications of stimulus-class and response covariation phenomena are profound.

Empirically Derived Expansions of the Stimulus and Response Concepts

As argued earlier, basic research work with ABA, as well as with TEAB, has led to an expanded view of behavior-control processes, and this view is remarkably similar to that outlined decades ago by B. F. Skinner (1938) and by J. R. Kantor (1920). Both theorists envisioned a paradigm in which behavior is a *complex* function of environmental events. In their arguments the term "function" was highlighted as a critical feature of one's theoretical understanding of behavior. A dictionary definition of function (Webster, 1975: "a thing that depends on and varies with something else") suggests a conception marked by regularities between and among events.

Within the three-term operant framework, individual behavior is explained and understood by functional events immediately preceding (discriminative stimuli) and following (reinforcement or punishment) the occurrence of behavior. The utility of this framework has been demonstrated numerous times in both the ABA and TEAB literature. A most familiar example in the ABA literature involves the enhancement of child prosocial behaviors. Specifically, B. L. Hopkins (1968) demonstrated the increase of social smiling of a young boy with the use of discriminative training and reinforcement. During walks in the school yard, the boy was given a piece of candy after smiling at passersby. Not surprisingly, the frequency of smiling in the context of meeting others increased substantially. Essentially, Hopkins demonstrated that a child's social smiling could be functionally controlled by events that preceded (discriminative stimuli) and followed (reinforcement) the occurrence of behavior.

Within the TEAB literature, a familiar application of the three-term operant framework involves the discriminative pecking of pigeons to different visual stimuli. Initially, a pigeon finds that pecking at a white light is followed by food. However, when the light is changed to green, pecking is no longer followed by food. Consequently, pecking at the light increases when the light is white and decreases when the light is green. The light color and the food in this case are the environmental events that functionally control the occurrence of pecking.

The usefulness and popularity of the three-term operant framework for explaining behavior has grown considerably over the years. Not unexpectedly, the topical areas involved have grown as well from an early emphasis on relatively simple issues (e.g., discriminative smiling in ABA, discriminative pecking in TEAB) to more complex behavioral phenomena (e.g., behavioral ecology in ABA, schedule-induced induction in TEAB). Additional to the increase in topics, an expansion of the basic three-term framework has been proposed. E. P. Willems (1974) suggested that a more ecological-systemic approach was needed in the field, an approach that not only included the three primary concepts but also included an examination of unintended "side effects" from behavioral interventions. The study of these "side effects" and subsequent expansion of the operant framework has focused on two of the three primary concepts, responses, and antecedent stimuli.

Expansion of the Response Concept

On the response side of the framework, investigators within ABA have documented that alterations in environment-behavior functional relationships may be accompanied by changes in the frequency of nontargeted responses. Basically, this research has shown that individual responses may not operate in a separate and discrete manner. Rather, individual responses may be interdependent in the sense that changes in frequency of one response may covary with the changes in frequency of another. For example, L. H. Epstein and colleagues (1974) found that a behavioral procedure for decreasing the frequency of inappropriate body movements in a schizophrenic child not only decreased the body movements but also increased the frequency of child toy play and verbal behaviors. Responses that initially appeared independent were actually interdependent with respect to the imposed behavioral procedure. This noted response covariation indicates that the behavioral unit influenced by Epstein and colleagues was not a discrete response but a more complex cluster of interdependent responses.

Although the organizational properties of the response-cluster phenomenon remains puzzling, this expansion of the response concept to include interdependent response clusters fits well within the operant framework. B. F. Skinner (1938) acknowledged that individual responses of an organism may form an interdependent set or class of responses as when members of the set are found to be functionally related to specific environmental contingencies. Additionally, members of the response class may or may not be topographically similar; overt similarity among the individual members of the response class is not a necessary requirement. What is important is that a systematic relationship between environmental contingencies and changes in the frequency of member responses be demonstrated.

Hence, the response covariation described in the ABA literature (e.g., Epstein, et al., 1974) appears very compatible with the operant framework. Response covariation is noted typically in cases where environmental contingencies are altered to change the frequency of some target response. These environmental changes are found to alter not only target responses but also nontarget behaviors. With respect to the environmental contingencies, the interdependent target and nontarget behavioral cluster appears to be the operant phenomenon Skinner called a response class. Although described by Skinner, the question of how individual responses become interdependent was not discussed.

We have described how investigators within TEAB and ABA have been conducting research aimed at describing the organizational properties of the response-class phenomenon. Unfortunately, none of the hypotheses concerning response covariation have generated much empirical backing. As L. M. Voeltz and I. M. Evans (1982) outlined in their review, functional linkages between and among an individual's responses cannot be explained as due to the governing influence of a common reinforcer, mediating autonomic respondent processes or sequential stimulus-response chains. However, an intriguing new conception of response covariation by W. Timberlake has been supported in laboratory studies. This conceptualization, known as behavior regulation (Timberlake, 1984), begins with the premise that free baseline levels of responding can be viewed as behavioral set points; free baseline responding represents a precontingency equilibrium condition of the organism. Therefore when a contingency is imposed on a response, the equilibrium set point of that response is disturbed. For example, a contingency schedule may be applied that limits access to food and reduces the frequency of eating behaviors to a level below the free baseline level. This imposed disequilibrium results in the organism altering responding of another behavior (for example, running) above its set point so that restoration of the equilibrium of the first response will be approached. In this way, two distinct responses may become linked, may be found to covary, since "the tendency to return to the previous level of one response must be expressed by changes in the other response" (Timberlake, 1984, p. 357). The phenomenon of response covariation, according to this perspective, may be the result of the individual's learning history and responses used to restore the equilibrium of other responses. Although preliminary, the behavior regulation conceptualization of response covariation indicates the continued interest within the field of behavior analysis in trying to understand the interdependence of behavior.

Expansion of the Stimulus Concept

Recently, ABA researchers have reported that events or situations that do not directly act on behavior (that is, do not serve as discriminative or reinforcing stimuli) nevertheless appear functionally related to the occurrence of behavior. In a correlational study concerning aversive interactions between mothers and children, R. G. Wahler (1980) found cases in which aversive maternal behavior was unrelated to the immediate stimuli provided by the child. Instead, aversive maternal behavior appeared to covary with coercive mother-adult interactions occurring earlier in the day. Maternal aversive behavior was found not to be a function of immediate and discrete stimuli but to be directly related to complex and temporally distant behavioral-environmental events. In a similar case, R. Forehead, J. Briener, R. J. McMahon, and G. Davies (1981) found that a behavioral strategy for decreasing aversive child behavior in the home was associated not only with a decrease in home aversive behavior but also with an increase in aversive behavior in school. Both the Wahler and Forehand, et al., studies suggest that temporally distant and complex events, events not included in the typical definition of discriminative stimuli, may influence the occurrence of behavior.

These temporally distant and complex events are anomalies to the traditional three-term operant framework, and they may be more appropriately classified as "setting factors" or "setting events." The concept of setting factors was described originally by J. R. Kantor (1959), and it referred to those situations that influenced the occurrence of stimulus-response relations previously learned through past organism-environment interactions (Wahler & Fox, 1981). These setting factors were conceptualized as complex and temporally distant behavioral-environmental conditions (e.g., water deprivation) that influenced behavioral patterns. S. W. Bijou and D. M. Baer (1961) then expanded the setting-factor to the setting-event concept by including environmental conditions and/or behavioral interactions which because they have occurred may influence current or later behavioral performance.

The setting-event concept is descriptive of the anomalies reported by Wahler (1980) and Forehand, et al. (1981), as well as the earlier described behavioral contrast and superstition phenomena (Fowler & Baer, 1981; Simon, Ayllon, & Milan, 1983. In all four studies, the occurrence of temporally distant and complex behavioral interactions was found to affect later responding. For Wahler, aversive adult interactions served as setting events for later mother-child aversive interactions, much the same as instructions and delayed reinforcer deliveries controlled children's sharing behavior in Fowler and Baer. In the Forehand, et al., study, extinction and punishment at home for aversive behavior served as a setting event for later aversive episodes at school, just as extinction caused a similar behavioral-contrast effect in the Simon, Ayllon, and Milan study.

TEAB investigators have documented still other ways in which complex behavioral-environmental conditions may influence discrete behavioral events. One such phenomenon, the matching law (Herrnstein, 1961), concerns the choices made by a subject when offered two or more concurrent schedules of reinforcement. Basically, this law indicates that the distribution of behavior between two or more schedules of reinforcement will be a direct ratio of the reinforcements obtained on each available schedule. For example, when faced with two schedules of food presentation, the second of which was offered twice as much food as the first, the subject will exert twice as much behavior (in either frequency or time) on the second schedule. As such, the matching law describes the effect that one schedule of reinforcement may have on behavior under another schedule of reinforcement. Although the matching law has been a topic of study for several years in the TEAB literature, only recently have its implications been extended to ABA. Myerson and Hale (1984) proposed that the behavioral results of the matching law could be of great value to applied investigators when attempting to decrease inappropriate behavior. Accordingly, inappropriate behavior should decrease in frequency and/or time if the individual is offered a richer schedule of reinforcement for some competing (and hopefully appropriate) behavior. Thus, to reduce disruptive classroom behavior of a child, the child could be offered praise for school work on a fairly rich schedule of reinforcement. Naturally, Myerson and Hale advise that such applied applications be studied more thoroughly prior to extended use so that possible complications of the natural environment be found.

As the above review indicates, investigators within TEAB and ABA have documented phenomena difficult to explain in terms of temporally immediate and discrete antecedent stimuli. But with a shift in the level of behavioral analysis from molecular to molar, an understanding of these phenomena emerges. Such a shift, permitting the study of covariations among molar as well as molecular events, has been previously described as a *behavioral systems* strategy (Wahler & Hann, 1986). As previously discussed, the strategy considers both a fine-grained view of responses and stimulus units plus more broadly construed units comprised of response and stimulus classes. An introduction to clinical child psychology from this strategic perspective would be primarily concerned with interdependencies between and among these units. Thus, when children behave in a deviant manner (e.g., chronic stealing), the deviant responses must be viewed within a context of other responses within that child's repertoire. Likewise, a mother's unfortunate use of threats or coddling must be seen as the figural parts of a repertoire context comprised of other ways she behaves. Furthermore, an understanding of how these response classes are maintained requires the interested clinician to examine intuitively obvious discriminative stimuli and the less apparent setting-event phenomena. Thus, a mother's threats leading to her child's noncompliance will yield a useful hypothesis on the maintenance issue. But her quarrels with her mother might also prove related to the likelihood of her threats and the child's noncompliance. This latter component of the stimulus class governing the mother's maladaptive child-care behavior will be crucial to the planning of a therapeutic intervention; that is, her threats are a function of the child's behavior and her quarrels with her own mother—a peculiar stimulus class indeed. The *art* of clinical child psychology as it is practiced from a behavioral systems perspective is a complex and often nonintuitive process.

Clinical Child Psychology

The most common psychological problems of childhood are antisocial and dependency behaviors. More than a third of the referrals to mental health centers are based on the child's antisocial or unduly aggressive actions such as fighting, temper outbursts, rule violations, stealing, and refusal to accept responsibilities (Roach, 1958). The same epidemiological studies show that dependency problems are next in referral frequency; these include phobias, separation fears, social withdrawal, and unfounded somatic complaints. Typically, the referrals are initiated by concerned adults (rather than the child) who voice their concerns in fairly global fashion. Fortunately, these ambiguous reports can readily be translated into specific events through self-report indices geared to the relevant adults—parents and teachers. Commonly used questionnaires are the Child Behavior Checklist (Achenbach, 1979), the Behavior Problem Checklist (Quay & Peterson, 1975), and the Connors Parent Rating Scale (Goyette, Conners, & Ulrich, 1978). Thus, the interbehavioral clinician will quickly obtain behavioral targets for more fine-grained observational assessment. However, it is important to realize the imperfect correspondence between these adult summary reports and observational findings on what the referred children actually do. Validity studies have shown good correspondence between parent checklist reports of child antisocial actions and observer reports of these behaviors in home settings (Hendricks, 1972; Patterson, 1974). But the studies also indicate a loose and sometimes poor correspondence between parent reports of child-dependency problems and the direct observational findings (Green, Beck, Forehand, & Vosk, 1983). In addition, some parent reporters are notoriously biased in their judgments of child deviance (Griest, Wells, & Forehand, 1979; Mash, Johnston, & Kovitz, 1983). The overall conclusion to be drawn from these studies must not only center on the obvious cautionary note with regard to ultimate targets of intervention; there is also an evident need to assess the parents who initiate the clinical referral. The latter need is central to an interbehavioral view of clinical work. When a child is referred for psychological problems, the clinician should be prepared to explain the importance of a broad-based approach to these problems. Although some of the parents' reports about child behavior will prove accurate, *other aspects may reflect the influence of stimuli extraneous to child behavior.*[1]

Interbehavioral clinicians are likely to follow the stimulus-class model in a pursuit of parent-referral descriptions. The stimulus-class concept, in line with our earlier arguments, presumes a functional equivalence among stimuli within sets comprising the family ecosystem. The sets are idiosyncratic to particular families and constitute cues or signals guiding each family member's behavior. Thus, a mother might respond aversively to her problem child after a variety of antecedent events. She is most likely to "snap" at her child if he or she whines, but she is also apt to behave in this fashion following an argument with her

1. One might note the convergence of interbehavioral and psychodynamic positions on this issue. Psychodynamists have long argued that a referral complaint is merely a "symptom" of a larger problem. While the two positions differ on the nature of this larger problem, they are in essential agreement on the initial conceptualization of referral complaints.

husband or some other significant adult (Paniccione & Wahler, 1986). Likewise, this same mother's summary report about her child's "aggression" could be determined by these disparate stimuli. She might describe her child as "demanding" because of the youngster's whining, nagging, and yelling; in addition, a mother's abrasive interchanges with her husband or mother could influence the nature of this report (Griest & Wells, 1983). The important feature of stimulus-class phenomena is seen in their puzzling composition. When an individual responds following the occurrence of a particular stimulus, one cannot assume that this stimulus, and those of topographic similarity, *causes* the response. Since most clinical work is correlational in nature, the caveat is crucial: the actual antecedent causal event might be quite different from that suspected on an intuitive basis.

As implied above, many parents who refer their children for clinical intervention are *overinclusive* in terms of the stimulus-class determinants of their concern as well as in their manner of responding to the problem child. The crucial aspect of this phenomenon centers on its potential inhibitory function with respect to clinical intervention. Suppose, for example, that the interbehavioral clinician decides to teach an abusive mother to use a time-out contingency following instances of her child's yelling. In order for such an intervention to "work," the mother would need to track the relevant stimuli (child yelling) and consistently apply time-out upon the occurrences. Yet, if child yelling is one component of an overinclusive stimulus class governing the mother's abuse, complications might arise. That is, her newly learned discipline skill would be performed in haphazard fashion if other stimuli in the class (e.g., arguments with spouse) influence her use of discipline. As we argued earlier, the stimulus-class model presumes a fairly broad-based approach to clinical assessment and intervention.

Before turning to a specific discussion of interbehavioral strategies on assessment and intervention, it will prove useful to highlight another previously discussed concept having to do with organizational features of the troubled child's behavior. Interbehavioral clinicians are likely to view child behavior as organized into *response classes* (see Kazdin's review, 1982). According to the concept, responses in a child's repertoire will display covariations suggesting the presence of functional classes. That is, the child's yelling, nagging, hitting, and noncompliance might be shown to covary over time, indicating a functional similarity among these responses. In other cases the covariations could be negative or inverse, pointing to an incompatibility between or among responses. Documented empirical examples of direct as well as inverse response covariations have been offered by R. G. Wahler (1975), P. S. Strain and D. Ezzell (1978), and A. Harris (1979).

The clinical utility of assessing response-class phenomena in troubled children is fairly clear. Some child problem behaviors constitute marked obstacles to therapeutic change, either because they occur outside the scope of adult surveillance (stealing) or because they are extraordinarily difficult to manage (explosive tantrum). However, should these response targets prove to covary with more readily changed responses in the child's repertoire, the possibility of *indirect* therapeutic change arises. Thus, R. G. Wahler and J. J. Fox (1980) discovered inverse correlations between oppositional children's rule violations and their solitary toy play. Then, in the anticipated intervention, the children's parents were taught to set contingencies designed to increase the rate of toy play. Results confirmed the functional incompatibility of these two responses; as toy play increased in frequency, rule violations decreased. Further experimental manipulations of the toy play contingency documented the functional relationships in all three children.

Clinical guidance from the response-class concept also applies to one's assessment of a parent's involvement in child behavior problems. When a mother is observed to engage her oppositional child in episodes of aversive confrontation, a clinician will wonder why she argues with the youngster instead of using some better means of dealing with the problem. The question of *why* is not only a stimulus-class issue because a mother's argument responses are likely to covary with other facets of her response repertoire. Thus, as Paniccione and Wahler (1986) showed, her aversive responses to child demands correlate with her confrontational dealings with spouse and other adults, as well as her self-reports of depression. When the clinician decides to help the mother shift her child argument responses to ignoring or a time-out or response-cost alternative, that professional will also consider her response covariations. Perhaps her depression and confrontations with adults are class members related to her child argument responses. If so, the targets of an upcoming therapeutic intervention would not be restricted to the mother's child-care behavior and she might also be helped to deal with these covarying parts of her response unit. Obviously, response-class phenomena, as well as stimulus-class phenomena, reflect keystone concepts in an interbehavioral approach to clinical work. As we shall see in the next two sections, this approach yields some useful assessment and intervention strategies.

Clinical Assessment

Response and Stimulus Conceptions

As expected from our previously discussed emphasis on molar as well as molecular conceptions of stimulus-response interactions, interbehavioral assessment is most useful in the planning of interventions when measurement is geared to both conceptual levels. The utility of such multilevel assessment is apparent in considering the troubled child's behavior, family members' behaviors, and the interactions between and among these events. The previously outlined term *class* (response or stimulus) will be used to designate a molar view of family events as opposed to a fine-grained picture obtained when the component members of a class are studied. Consider the assessment issues presented when a child's deviant behaviors are examined as particular responses and as response classes. Loeber and Schmaling (in press) have demonstrated the importance of a distinction between overt and covert forms of child opposition problems. Overtly oppositional children are, by definition, openly confrontive with their parents as seen in refusals to comply with instructions, complaints, threats, and physical harassment. Covertly oppositional children, while they are also non-compliant, act so in reference to rules rather than instructions. Because they are apt to comply with parental commands, these children do not present immediate discipline problems. But, once outside the scope of parental surveillance, the covertly oppositional youngster will disobey rules against stealing, substance use, truancy, and property destruction.

Overtly oppositional children can be assessed in fine-grained fashion through direct observation by the children's parents and professional observers. By noting the children's specific means of opposing parental instructions (e.g., nagging, whining), intervention targets are presented. On the other hand, covertly oppositional children do not display their deviant behaviors in the presence of adults and, thus, cannot be assessed in detailed fashion. Instead, the observer must rely on after-the-fact indices of the covert transgressions (e.g., when a teacher reports a child's school absence; when a parent smells smoke on the child's breath). In effect, the assessor must assume that the chosen index is part of the targeted *class* of covert opposition. Although the index is a specific behavior, the intent behind its measurement is not simply to alter that behavior. It is hoped that when the index response changes there will be accompanying changes in the more important components of the covert response class. This hope has some empirical backing in reference to the covert problems of stealing (Patterson, Reid, Jones, & Conger, 1975; Reid & Hendricks, 1973). As long as a parent can correctly define and then punish the stealing index (having an article not belonging to him or her), occurrences of the index as well as reports of the covert violation by community members decrease in frequency.

The importance of considering specific child problem behaviors as members of molar response classes is also seen in studies of children's noncompliance with parental instructions. A variety of molecular problem behaviors, such as tantrums and unfounded fear reactions, covary inversely with the children's opposition to parental instructions. In line with the research findings of Russo, Cataldo, and Cushing (1981), noncompliance seems to be a keystone response in the repertoires of troubled children. Unfortunately, most parents view child compliance in an abstract sense as contrary to their hopes for eventual child independence. Russo and colleagues (1981) showed that this expectation is unfounded at least when a child's chronic noncompliance is considered. When these oppositional children become more compliant with parental instructions, a number of desirable options become available to the children (also see Patterson, 1982, p. 250).

The clinical assessment implications of response-class phenomena in troubled children have been reviewed elsewhere by Wahler and Fox (1981) and by Kazdin (1982). By now, a fairly large body of empirical data support the utility of considering the complete repertoires of these children rather than the relevant deviant responses alone. Whatever the governing principles of response-class organization (e.g., Timberlake, 1984), it is clear that the clinician's knowledge of such organizational features can be a valuable aid in the planning of interventions.

In considering family members' reactions to the troubled child's behavior, molar as well as molecular conceptions of these individuals' behaviors continue to be useful. Thus far, response-class research in this area has been restricted to parental reactions to the child, mothers in particular. While family members' reactions are appropriately considered on the stimulus side of child behavior problems, family members are also considered as intervention targets and, thus, a response perspective is equally important. A mother's reactions to her troubled child appear critical in two categories: (a) her responses directed to the child's deviant and adaptive behaviors; (b) her summary judgments about the child's problems. In reference to the first issue, an important problem in implementing therapeutic change within families has to do with the troubled mother's tendency to react aversively to her "problem" child. Although these reactions are largely determined by the child's deviant behaviors, there are data suggesting that her aversive child-care responses covary with other aspects of her own repertoire. Thus, Patterson (1982, pp. 192–96) has presented correlational data pointing to an "irritability" characteristic of troubled mothers. Irritability means that these mothers were likely to continue their aversive reactions to their children regardless of how the children behaved. Likewise, these mothers were apt to start a coercive exchange with their children even if the youngsters were behaving in a positive manner. In support of Patterson's findings, Pannicione and Wahler (1985) discovered that mothers' self-reports of depression covaried with their probabilities of reacting aversively to child behavior. The relevance of such response styles with troubled mothers is similar to that cited in our earlier discussion of keystone responses in the troubled child's repertoire. If indeed there is a traitlike facet of maladaptive maternal care, its identification through careful measurement ought to yield more options when intervention strategies are considered.

A troubled mother's summary judgments about her problem child also show some interesting response-class connections. Before describing these connections we should first point out the critical role of a parent's summary judgments in child development. Such judgments are the initial bases for a clinical referral as well as other important considerations with respect to the child's welfare (e.g., whether or not the child is allowed to go camping or play sports). Thus, when a mother offers a judgment about her child, one would hope that this report is determined by what the child does or does not do. Unfortunately, the available evidence suggests some possible covariations between these maternal judgments and other components of her response repertoire. Similar to the "irritability" class (Patterson, 1982), a mother's judgments can be predicted by what that mother says about her depressed mood (Griest, Wells, & Forehand, 1978; Paniccione & Wahler, 1986). As her feelings of depression increase, so does the tendency to describe her child as deviant. Not surprisingly, mothers who admit to pronounced depressive moods are also apt to experience performance difficulties when intervention strategies are implemented (McMahan, Forehand, Griest, & Wells, 1981).

Although the evidence reviewed above is appropriately conceptualized on the response side of a clinical assessment paradigm, these data apply to stimulus conceptions as well. The covariation between a mother's judgments about her child and her depressed mood appears related to a global class of stimuli. This class, broadly conceived, includes the actions of her child (aversive stimuli such as nagging) and the actions of adults in her family and community (aversive stimuli such as quarrels with husband). In the study by Panaccione and Wahler (1986), correlational analyses showed these child and adult aversive stimuli to be reasonably good predictors of maternal depression and maternal judgments of child deviance. Likewise, R. G. Wahler and M. G. Graves (1983) found the same stimulus class associated with a troubled mother's negative reactions to her problem child. The important factor evident in all of the previously reviewed studies centers on the multidetermined nature of any targeted response or stimulus. For example, when a troubled mother is observed to react angrily to her oppositional child, one cannot assume that her anger response is a simple function of what the child has done (Wahler & Graves, 1983), nor can one use a mother's clearly stated concern about her child's deviance as an infallible index of child behavior. Troubled mothers are apt to respond to broad, *overinclusive* stimulus classes.

Clinical research studies of stimulus-class phenomena affecting child behavior have yet to be conducted. However, based on field studies with normal children there is good reason to believe that children are also subject to the influence of overinclusive stimulus classes. For example, S. A. Fowler and D. M. Baer (1981) demonstrated this form of stimulus control with preschool children in free-play settings. The children were first instructed to share toys with their peers and then were reinforced with points for doing so in a morning preschool play setting. Following this operation, the point reinforcers were delayed until an afternoon time, but they were still contingent on sharing responses in the morning setting. This done, the children's sharing in an afternoon free-play setting increased in frequency, even though the point deliveries had nothing to do with this later setting. Thus, the instructions to share plus the noncontingent reinforcers controlled child behaviors that were actually unrelated to one another—just as the troubled mothers were influenced by child irrelevant stimuli.

Based on the above study, one might presume that a troubled child's deviant relationships with family members might be influenced by stimuli other than those emanating from the problem relationship. Thus, an oppositional child's tendency to oppose maternal instructions could be determined by mother's behavior *and* the child's recent interactions with peers. The temporally immediate stimuli shown to govern a troubled child's deviant behavior are probably not the complete class influencing that child's behavior. Just as the behavior of troubled mothers is often governed by overinclusive stimulus classes, troubled children are likely to behave in kind.

Practical Implications of Response- and Stimulus-Class Phenomena

The conceptual arguments presented above can be translated in specific assessment procedures, geared to the troubled child and key family members— the child's mother in particular. In line with our emphasis on both molar and molecular views of stimuli and responses, appropriate measures include parent and child summary reports of problems as well as more detailed frequency counts sampling these problem events. On the molar side of assessment, self-report rating scales such as the Child Behavior Checklist (Achenbach, 1979) and the Beck Depression Inventory (Beck, 1970) will yield reliable parental reports on specific child problems and more general parental problems. Similar, psychometrically sound rating scales for the child's use are not as available. To our knowledge there are no scales for assessing child reports on specific parent problems, although a child version of the Beck Depression Inventory (Kovacs, 1980) has proven to be reliable for elementary school-age children. If the clinician has sampled these summary reports by parents and the target child, a useful sort of comparison can then be initiated between the summary reports and the later described frequency counts reflecting the actual behaviors of these people. Thus, a convergence between parental reports of deviant child withdrawal and observational counts of infrequent child social interaction would suggest a fairly straightforward intervention. A lack of convergence, on the other hand, would require further examination of covariations among the obtained measures (e.g., inspections of parental depression reports and parental child-behavior reports). Before discussing these class possibilities, let us examine some strategies in obtaining the molecular measures.

Based on parent summary reports of child-behavior problems and interview-based elaborations of these reports, it becomes feasible to define concrete instances of any child problem (see Wahler & Cormier, 1970). As long as the instances are specific and observable (e.g., having an item not belonging to him or her; teasing his or her little brother), an observer ought to be able to monitor and record occurrences in a dependable manner. Basically two formats have been used in recording strategy (after Patterson, 1982, pp. 41–65). The first format is the sampling of those problem behaviors likely to occur in a parent's presence. These "overt" behaviors such as separation protests, clinging, demands, noncompliance, and temper outbursts can be noted by the parent in some time reference (e.g., 30-minute period). By the same token, the parent's self-observed reactions to these child responses (demands or reasoning) as well as parental provocation (instructions or irritable approaches) could be recorded in the same time period. However, since this part of the recording strategy stretches the limits of parent objectivity, a neutral party is typically used to obtain information on parental responses to the child. In addition, such third-party assessment can serve as a reliability check on all facets of the parents' recording.

The second format involves monitoring by the parent, in after-the-fact format, those child problem behaviors likely to occur outside parent presence. "Covert" actions, such as leaving school, property destruction, and substance abuse, can be sampled by a parent if that adult is willing to institute and maintain a communication network with other people who interact with the child (teachers, extended family). Defining a covert problem is also a critical part of the surveillance process because the parent will not have first-hand knowledge of the problem occurrence. In essence, the parent must define an occurrence as *after-the-fact evidence regardless of the child's explanation* (e.g., teacher report of child fighting, child failing to bring homework home, parent smelling smoke on child). While this procedure is unfair in a legal sense, its one-sided application is critical to the success of later intervention (see Reid & Hendricks, 1973).

In the same spirit by which covert child problems are monitored, it is possible to keep track of parental problems occurring outside the parent-child dyad. As long as the clinical interviewer shifts a parent's focus to potential marital disputes and extrafamily aversive encounters, these problem episodes can also be defined in a concrete manner.

Given that a clinician has access to sets of molar and molecular data on parent and child, some systematic class comparisons ought to be pursued. Those likely to yield useful information are outlined below.

1. *Child response classes*. If daily records of child overt and covert problem responses are obtained, it is possible to inspect covariations between various response combinations following R. G. Wahler and J. J. Fox (1980). Thus, a child's property destruction might be shown to covary with instances of his or her noncompliance with parental instructions. In addition, some of the child's self-reports (e.g., depression) might also covary with these molecular responses.

2. *Parent response classes*. The response covariation tactic can again be followed in reference to a parent's behavior "style." Most important in this respect are potential covariations between frequency counts of parental approaches, instructions, and reactions to child behavior and that parent's summary reports of depression, anxiety, and views held by the parent about the child (global views of child intent, global assessment of child deviance). Thus, a mother's marked use of vaguely stated instructions could covary with her frequently voiced reports about the child's "playing dumb."

3. *Stimulus classes for parent responses*. In this case the covariations of interest concern parent responses (molar or molecular) and indices of stimuli within the parent's family and community. The obvious and relevant stimuli ought to be represented by the molecular indices of child behavior, in particular those behaviors considered deviant. However, since troubled mothers tend to be influenced by overinclusive stimulus classes, child irrelevant stimuli could also covary with the mother's child-care behaviors. Thus, a mother's use of explanation

following her child's demands might covary with her self-report indices reflecting abrasive encounters with her husband.

4. *Stimulus classes for child responses*. While these inspections have yet to be subjected to research analyses, we suspect that troubled children are also influenced by overinclusive stimulus classes. For example, a molar index of the child's negative peer interactions could be found to covary with his or her problem interaction involving a parent.

Although the above analyses of obtained assessment data could be conducted with research rigor, our intention is to foster clinical application. In our day-to-day service delivery work, the previously discussed associations between measures are viewed in "eyeball" comparisons through simple graphing of the data. The important point to stress is that intervention can now be viewed as a variety of options, ranging from the familiar use of contracting and time-out to more complex means of attenuating the influence of overinclusive stimulus classes. We turn now to a look at these options.

Clinical Intervention

Contingency Management

The planning and implementation of direct changes in parent-child interactions is a central feature of the interbehavioral strategy. This familiar approach, often described as "parent training" (see Dangel & Polster, 1984), is aimed at modifying associations between specific child responses and specific parent responses (the latter viewed as stimuli). Because the literature is replete with research-documented examples of the modifications and their functional impact, there is little need for an extensive review here. Suffice it to say that the modifications are guided by the three-term operant contingency in which parents are taught to recognize how their behaviors can and do serve discriminative and reinforcing functions for deviant child behavior. Given this "surveillance" training, the parents are then taught to replace these maladaptive contingencies with new ways of relating to their children. The new ways, typically entailing parental ignoring, praise, time-out, and material rewards are discussed with both parent and child and then practiced until the parent meets some criterion performance.

Although contingency management procedures are always designed to alter some designated behavior, clinical research has also shown the value of this strategy in producing predictable *indirect* effects. The concept of indirect therapeutic change is, of course, tied to previously reviewed interbehavioral assumptions regarding the organizational properties of an individual's response repertoire. Successful contingency management interventions will sometimes result in two types of collateral change in nontargeted responses (see Wahler & Fox, 1980) and, thus, the following indirect change possibilities should be considered.

Interrupting sequential patterns of maladaptive interaction. Patterson (1982, pp. 275–80) has presented data to show that some response-class phenomena are due to dependable linkages in parent-child interaction. These functional linkages begin with a mildly aversive response by one member of the dyad and lead in sequence to other aversive exchanges. While the early exchanges might not constitute intervention targets (e.g., child nag), the later exchanges are often significant clinical problems (e.g., child temper outburst or parent hitting child). The importance of detecting such sequential patterns obviously centers on the timing of a contingency management target. Rather than waiting for later, highly relevant targets of the pattern, a more effective intervention would entail stopping the pattern during its early sequential steps. Applications of this intervention strategy are seen in child-abuse problems (see Reid, 1984) and may also apply to child-dependency problems such as separation anxiety (see Wahler & Dumas, 1985). In the former case, physical abuse by a parent usually appears as the end product of a sequential pattern initiated through innocuous but irritating parent-child exchanges. In the latter case, a child's hysterical refusal to leave a parent (e.g., on the way to school) will often begin with parent-child discussions about the child's somatic complaints. Now, while there are data to support contingency management interventions with such "early warning" parent-child exchanges, the clinician must proceed with caution. In our experience, parents will readily grasp the rationale of this intervention strategy but find the procedure unduly harsh given the child offense (e.g., complaining of a stomachache). Even when assessment data repeatedly show the sequential escalation, some parents are understandably reluctant to proceed with the recommended contingency step.

Contingency management of "keystone" responses. When two or more responses in a child's or parent's repertoire are shown to covary, but no sequential patterning is evident, there is still reason to pursue indirect contingency management. As we noted at the beginning of this chapter, the organizational properties of *most* response covariation phenomena have yet to be understood (see Voeltz & Evans, 1982). Some clinical research studies indicate that predictable changes may occur in children's intercorrelated deviant actions when one response in the cluster is modified (see Kazdin's 1982 review). Although the composition of these clusters or classes may be idiosyncratic to each troubled child, some common classes are suggested. Thus, in Wahler and Fox (1980) three conduct-disordered children were shown to reduce the frequencies of their oppositional behaviors following a successful contingency intervention geared to increasing frequencies of their solitary play. Likewise, Voeltz and Evans (1982) cited several empirical studies in which children's increased compliance with adult instructions served as a keystone intervention—leading to reductions in the children's aggressive responses.

Thus far, little research work has been devoted to intervention possibilities with parent-response classes. For example, Pannicione and Wahler (1986) found mothers' self-reports of depression to covary with their aversive reactions to their children. Unfortunately, the molar self-report response in this cluster does not lend itself to any simple contingency management intervention. A pursuit of such keystone response factors in a parent's child-care behavior ought to follow the same strategy found useful with children—correlational analyses of molecular parent responses. Parents obviously do more than discipline and praise their children in a day-to-day household routine. Some of these overlooked parent behaviors (recreational reading, watching television) might well covary with the critical child-care responses.

Stimulus-Class Modifications

When a parent and child change their response styles with respect to one another, it seems reasonable to expect changes in each person's stimulus values. That is, when a mother uses her newly discovered contingency management procedures, her stimulus function for the child ought to change. If her previous function was to set the occasion for child avoidance or antagonism, her new function ought to produce different child reactions—ideally affection and pro-social interest. Likewise, the child's stimulus value for the mother should become positive and no longer evoke an earlier maladaptive child-care pattern. In effect, the two parties ought to like and enjoy each other's company after a successful contingency management intervention.

The above speculations presuppose some degree of generalization in specifically modified stimulus properties of parent and child. The generalization assumption is important because of previously discussed findings indicating that troubled mothers (and perhaps their children) may be influenced by *overinclusive* stimulus classes. One may recall that these findings portrayed some troubled mothers as behaving in maladaptive ways toward their children in the absence of relevant child-produced stimuli. Of course, the "relevant" stimuli for a mother's maladaptive child care should be comprised of the youngster's deviant actions. When these cues change through contingency management, one would hope that a mother's complete class of maladaptive reactions to her child will also change.

Available data suggest that generalized stimulus-class changes will occur with both mother and child after contingency management. Wahler (1969) assessed the reinforcement value of maternal priaise before and after teaching the mothers a time-out procedure for their oppositional children. Time-out applications by the mothers decreased the children's oppositional actions and *increased* the power of praise when used by the mothers in a laboratory setting. In effect, maternal praise was more effective in altering the children's laboratory play after the mothers had mastered their home-based use of time-out. Thus, the stimulus class presented by mothers not only changed in cue function (now setting the occasion for child compliance); the class also acquired new reinforcement value for the children. Patterson and Fleischman (1979) reviewed similar generalization outcomes in reference to children's stimulus-class functions for mothers. After clinic-referred mothers were effective in reducing their problem children's opposition, the mothers' global ratings of their youngsters shifted from negative to positive. The mothers enjoyed their children more after successful contingency management and also reported themselves to be less depressed.

Unfortunately, other studies show an absence of generalized stimulus-class changes following successful contingency management (see review by Griest & Wells, 1983). Thus, Forehand, Wells, and Griest (1980) taught clinic-referred mothers to produce significant reductions in their oppositional children's problem behaviors. However, when the mothers were asked to describe the observed changes they tended to negate the improvements. Likewise, Wahler and Afton (1980) found that some troubled mothers who produced successful change in their problem children continued to provide negative blame-oriented evaluations of the children. According to Wells' (1981) review of these anomalies, some parents' judgments about their children's behavior are based on parental "maladjustment." That is, parents who are under duress from extrachild problems (e.g., marital strife, social isolation) are apt to be more responsive to these problems than they are to child-rearing issues. Wells' "maladjusted" mother fits our criteria of mothers who are chronically influenced by overinclusive stimulus classes. Since these mothers' reactions to their children seem partly determined by extrachild problems, it is unlikely that they will consistently apply the attention and discipline needed to maintain the therapeutic benefits of contingency management. As two studies have shown, contingency management "failure cases" are marked by conflict between the mother and other adults, the absence of supportive relationships for the mother, and socioeconomic disadvantage (Dumas & Wahler, 1983; Webster-Stratton, 1985).

Troubled mothers whose child-care actions are governed by overinclusive stimulus classes also demonstrate peculiar summary reports. When these mothers are asked to define their biased child-behavior reports they are apt to offer little information. The reports tend to be comprised of a small number of referents compared to those offered by other, less troubled mothers (Wahler & Afton, 1980; Wahler & Hann, 1986). In the latter study, conversations between clinic-referred mothers and their parent trainers, friends, and kinfolk were tape-recorded and analyzed. Across the board, multistressed mothers (those with extrachild problems) communicated less information in their conversational reports about child problems than did singularly stressed mothers (those with child interaction problems only). Typically, the former mothers would describe their children in global terms and tend to use these same terms in repetitive fashion.

We suspect that a multistressed mother's conservative or narrow definition of child problem behavior might determine her overinclusive reactions to her child. If the mother's response definition is narrow in composition, she is unlikely to pay much attention to her stimulus field. Although her child-directed responses are governed by a wide range of stimuli, she is apt to attend to a selective subset of this overinclusive class. Thus, when she snaps at her child after returning from an aversive encounter with her sister, her report about the child interchange problem will not include the contextual exchange with the sister. Her handicap in child-care strategy is obvious if this assumption is correct. Regardless of how accurately she tracks her child in an effort to deal with the parenting problem, she will still be detrimentally influenced by the contextual stimuli. Until she attends to the larger picture of stimulus determinants, her capacity to deal constructively with the parenting problem is limited. Presumably, then, some means of expanding the mother's definition of deviance ought to affect her attentional framework. If she comes to view her contextual problems as part of her child relationship problems, she might also become more resourceful in handling these latter problems. In effect, she will "screen out" or categorize her contextual problems as separate from her child relationship problems. This selective focus ought to foster her use of child management procedures in day-to-day reactions to her child. In terms of observer-training strategies, she will become more reliable in coding child behavior because she discriminates these stimuli from other environmental events. Given her dependable coding of child behavior as separate from other stimuli in her life, this newly educated mother ought to use her education wisely. She would be expected to respond to her child solely on the basis of what her child does and does not do—a condition ideally suited for effective handling of child relationship problems.

Recently, Wahler and Dumas (1985) described a means of helping troubled mothers to expand their response definitions of child deviance. The procedure, called "mand review," is a conversational supplement to contingency management in which the parent trainer probes the referents of a mother's observational report.[2] Probes such as asking for greater detail and suggesting that additional referents might belong in the report are employed by the parent trainer in weekly dialog sessions. Thus, when a mother describes how her demanding child "takes over" by constantly interrupting her, the parent trainer will ask her to expand that report in a variety of ways. Some of these queries may direct the mother to explore details (e.g., what else was happening?) and other queries might direct her to compare the episode to other demanding episodes in her life (e.g., is that similar to what your husband did to you last week?). Wahler and Dumas (1985) found that clinic-referred multistressed mothers gradually expanded the information content of their reports as this sort of dialog continued over weeks. In addition, the home-based observation data showed that the mothers continued to apply their previously learned contingency management skills over the course of their dialog sessions. More to the point, Wahler, Sansbury, Bender, and Bryant (1985) found an association between mothers' report expansions and their more creative solutions to hypothetical child-rearing problems.

The previously described treatment strategy for troubled mothers suggests that the composition of overinclusive stimulus classes can be altered without pro-

2. Although contingency management procedures direct a mother to narrow her observational reports about child behavior, mand review procedures are geared in an opposite direction. We view the latter procedures as a *supplement* to contingency management. Although a mother formulates specific targets for contingency management, the parent trainer will also want her to talk about her original definitions and then to expand these definitions through the conversational shaping procedures of mand review.

ducing physical change in the mothers' environments. If a mother's redefinition of her observational report categories can attenuate her responsiveness to child irrelevant stimuli (e.g., arguments with spouse), the importance of attentional processes is highlighted. Evidently, the organizational properties of a stimulus class depend more on selective attention than reinforcement contingencies. A multistressed mother's reactions to her problem child's behavior sometimes has little to do with how that child consequated her reactions. On these occasions she appears to scan her stimulus field in selective fashion, attending to her reactions to prior events as she also attempts to focus on what her child is doing and saying. Under these conditions, she could hardly be expected to behave in any systematic or consistent manner in reference to her child. But when she changes her observational report categories through the sorts of conversation outlined earlier, she may also change her attentional operations. Even though the child irrelevant coercive experiences continue to occur, these mothers seem to "be done with them" once the experiences are over. Rather than dwelling on the historical context, she attends selectively and appropriately to the task at hand—namely, the current relationship with her child.

The Practicing Interbehavioral Clinician

Clinical child psychology from an interbehavioral perspective clearly fits within the general framework of behavior therapy or behavior modification. The interbehavioral clinician is concerned with observable events and is likely to interpret these events within the conceptual guidelines of operant and respondent learning theories. But while this clinician is constrained by a reliance on observable events, these constraints do not necessarily include the strict guidelines of learning theory. As J. R. Kantor noted in the first chapter of this book, "Since clinical work concerns complaints about interbehavior, the clinician can concentrate upon the activities of integral individuals and reject guidance from traditional theoretical abstractions." In our opinion, the term "integral individuals" refers to the behavioral systems strategy outlined earlier: individuals are best understood in reference to their molecular responses and the molar covariations among these responses and stimuli comprising environments. Sometimes these covariations are understandable within the principles of operant and respondent learning theories and sometimes they are not. If a particular covariation does not make theoretical sense (e.g., a mother's aversive response to her child following some unrelated encounter between the mother and another adult), the interbehavioral clinician will hardly be surprised. In essence, this lack of surprise means that this clinician is primarily concerned with a developing picture of event covariations, regardless of the form taken by these covariations. This well describes the interbehavioral clinician in actual practice.

We have been impressed with the "freewheeling" style of interbehavioral clinicians as they converse with their clients. During contingency management training, these clincians are systematic and laborious in their exchanges with troubled mothers and children. But once the management lessons are learned, the course of discussion is more difficult to follow. Clinician and mother seem to be following a systematic train of discourse, but the rules of this discourse are not evident on the basis of any general theory of therapy. Until the observer knows something about covariations comprising stimulus and response classes relevant to the mother and the child, the logic of clinician reactions to mother descriptions is hard to follow. Given a knowledge of the correlational "rules," however, the discourse is relatively easy to follow. A grasp of these correlationally derived rules is perhaps the keystone skill requirement for interbehavioral therapeutic work. A competent interbehavioral clinician must be well grounded in operant and classical conditioning principles. In addition to these conceptual guidelines, that clinician must become competent in the derivation of response- and stimulus-class principles idiosyncratic to the client. As we have attempted to argue, this latter strategy is the hallmark of interbehavioral clinical psychology.

References

Achenbach, T. M. 1979. Psychopathology of childhood: Research problems and issues. *Journal of Consulting and Clinical Psychology* 46: 759–76.

Beck, A. T. 1970. *Depression: Causes and treatment*. Philadelphia: University of Pennsylvania Press.

Bernstein, D. J., and E. B. Ebbesen. 1976. Reinforcement and substitution in humans: A multiple-response analysis. *Journal of the Experimental Analysis of Behavior* 30: 243–53.

Bijou, S. W., and D. M. Baer. 1961. *Child Development I: A systematic and empirical theory*. Englewood Cliffs, N.J.: Prentice-Hall.

Dangel, R. F., and R. A. Polster. (Eds.) 1984. *Parent training*. New York: Guilford Press.

Dumas, J. E., and R. G. Wahler. 1983. Predicators of treatment outcome in parent training: Mother insularity and socioeconomic disadvantage. *Behavioral Assessment* 5: 301–13.

Epstein, L. H., L. A. Doke, T. E. Sajwaj, S. Sorrell, and B. Rimner. 1974. Generality and side effects of overcorrection. *Journal of Applied Behavior Analysis* 7: 185–90.

Forehand, R., J. Briener, R. J. McNahan, and G. Davies. 1981. Predictors of cross setting behavior change in treatment of child problems. *Journal of Behavior Therapy and Experimental Psychiatry* 12: 311–13.

Forehand, R., K Wells, and D. Griest. 1980. An examination of the social validity of a parent training program. *Behavior Therapy* 11: 488–502.

Fowler, S. A., and D. M. Baer. 1981. Do I have to be good all day? The timing of delayed reinforcement as a factor in generalization. *Journal of Applied Behavior Analysis* 14: 14–24.

Goyette, C. H., C. K. Conners, and R. F. Ulrich. 1978. Normative data on revised Conners Parent and Teacher Rating Scales. *Journal of Abnormal Child Psychology* 6: 221–36.

Green, K. D., S. J. Beck, R. Forehand, and B. Vosk. 1983. Validity of teacher nominations of child behavior problems. *Journal of Abnormal Child Psychology.*

Griest, D. L., and K. C. Wells. 1983. Behavioral family therapy with conduct disorders in children. *Behavior Therapy* 14: 37–53.

Griest, D. L., K. C. Wells, and R. Forehand. 1979. An examination of predictors of maternal perceptions of maladjustment in clinic-referred children. *Journal of Abnormal Psychology* 88: 277–81.

Harris, A. 1979. An empirical test of the situation specificity/consistency of aggressive behavior. *Child Behavior Therapy* 1: 257–70.

Hendricks, A. F. C. J. 1972. Reported versus observed deviance. Unpublished manuscript, University of Nymegen, Netherlands.

Herrnstein, R. J. 1961. Relative and absolute strength of response as a function of frequency of reinforcement. *Journal of the Experimental Analysis of Behavior* 4: 267–72.

Herrnstein, R. J. and P. N. Hineline. 1966. Negative reinforcement as shock-frequency reduction. *Journal of the Experimental Analysis of Behavior* 19: 361–67.

Hopkins, B. L. 1968. Effects of candy and social reinforcement, instructions, and reinforcement schedule learning on the modification and maintenance of smiling. *Journal of Applied Behavior Analysis* 1: 121–29.

Kantor, J. R. 1920. Suggestions toward a scientific interpretation of perception. *Psychological Review* 27: 191–216.

Kantor, J. R. 1959. *Interbehavioral psychology*. Granville, Ohio: Principia Press.

Kazdin, A. E. 1982. Symptom substitution, generalization, and response covariation: Implications for psychotherapy outcomes. *Psychological Bulletin* 81: 349–65.

Kovacs, M. 1980. Rating scales to assess depression in school age children. *Acta Paedopsychiatrica* 46: 305–15.

Lambert, J. V., P. J. Bersh, P. M. Hineline, and G. A. Smith. 1973. Avoidance conditioning with shock contingent upon the avoidance response. *Journal of the Experimental Analysis of Behavior* 19: 361–67.

Loeber, R., and K. B. Schmaling. In press. Empirical evidence for overt and covert patterns of antisocial conduct problems. *Journal of Abnormal Child Psychology.*

McKearney, J. W., and J. E. Barrett, 1975. Punished behavior: Increases in responding after d-amphetamine. *Psychopharmacologia*, 41: 23–26.

McMahon, R. J., R. Forehand, D. L. Griest, and K. C. Wells. 1981. Who drops out of therapy during parent behavior training? *Behavioral Counseling Quarterly* 1: 79–85.

Michael, J. 1982. Distinguishing between discriminative and motivational functions of stimuli. *Journal of the Experimental Analysis of Behavior* 57: 149–55.

Morris, E. K., S. T. Higgins, and W. K. Bickel. 1982a. Comments on cognitive science in the experimental analysis of behavior. *Journal of Applied Behavior Analysis* 13: 23–39.

Morris, E. K., S. T. Higgins, and W. K. Bickel. 1982b. The influence of Kantor's interbehavioral psychology on behavior analysis. *The Behavior Analyst* 5: 158–73.

Myerson, J., and S. Hall. 1984. Practical implications of the matching law. *Journal of Applied Behavior Analysis* 17: 367–80.

O'Leary, K. D., and R. E. Emery. 1984. Marital discord and child behavior problems.

In M. D. Levine and P. Satz (Eds.), *Developmental variation and dysfunction*. New York: Academic Press.

Paniccione, V. F., and R. G. Wahler. 1986. Child behavior, maternal depression and social coercion as factors in the quality of child care. *Journal of Abnormal Child Psychology* 14:263–78.

Patterson, G. R. 1974. Interventions for boys with conduct problems: Multiple settings, treatments and criteria. *Journal of Consulting and Clinical Psychology* 42: 471–81.

Patterson, G. R. 1982. *Coercive family process*. Eugene, Ore.: Castalia Press.

Patterson, G. R., and M. J. Fleischman. 1979. Maintenance of treatment effects: Some considerations concerning family systems and follow-up data. *Behavior Therapy* 10: 168–85.

Patterson, G. R., J. B. Reid, R. R. Jones, and R. E. Conger. 1975. *A social learning approach to family intervention. Vol 1: Families with aggressive children*. Eugene, Ore.: Castalia Press.

Quay, H. C. and D. R. Peterson. 1975. Manual for the *Behavioral Problem Checklist*. Unpublished manuscript, University of Miami, Miami, Florida.

Reid, J. B. 1984. Social-interactional patterns in families of abused and nonabused children. In C. John Waxler, M. Cummings, and M. Rodke-Yarrow (Eds.), *Social and biological origin of altruism and aggression*. Boston, Mass.: Cambridge Press.

Reid, J. B., and A. F. C. J. Hendricks. 1973. A preliminary analysis of the effectiveness of direct home intervention for treatment of predelinquent boys who steal. In L. Hamerlynck, L. Handy, and E. Mash (Eds.), *Behavior therapy: Methodology, concepts, and practice*. Champaign, Ill.: Research Press.

Rescorla, R. A., and R. L. Solomon. 1967. Two-process learning theory: Relationships between Pavlovian conditioning and instrumental learning. *Psychological Review*, 74: 151–82.

Reynolds, G. S. 1961. Attention in the pigeon. *Journal of the Experimental Analysis of Behavior* 4: 203–08.

Roach, J. L. 1958. Some social-psychological characteristics of child guidance clinic caseloads. *Journal of Consulting Psychology* 22: 183–86.

Rogers-Warren, A. and S. F. Warren. (Eds.). 1977. *Ecological perspectives in behavior analysis*. Baltimore: University Park Press.

Russo, D. C., M. F. Cataldo, and P. J. Cushing. 1981. Compliance training and behavioral covariation in the treatment of multiple behavioral in the treatment of multiple behavior problems. *Journal of Applied Behavior Analysis* 14 (3): 209–22.

Simon, S. J., T. Ayllon, and M. A. Milan. 1982. Behavioral compensation: Contrast-like effects in the classroom. *Behavior Modification* 6: 407–20.

Sizemore, O. J., and K. A. Lattal. 1977. Dependency, temporal contiguity, and response-independent reinforcement. *Journal of the Experimental Analysis of Behavior* 27: 119–25.

Skinner, B. F. 1938. *The behavior of organisms*. New York: Appleton-Century-Crofts.

Skinner, B. F. 1953. *Science and human behavior*. New York: Macmillan.

Strain, P. S. and D. Ezzell. 1978. The sequence and distribution of behavioral disordered adolescents' disruptive/inappropriate behaviors: An observational study in a residential setting. *Behavior Modification* 2: 403–25.

Timberlake, W. (1984). Behavior regulation and learned performance: Some misapprehensions and disagreements. *Journal of the Experimental Analysis of Behavior* 41: 355–75.

Ullmann, L. P. and L. Krasner. (Eds.). 1965. *Case studies in behavior modification.* New York: Holt, Reinhart & Winston, pp. 1–63.

Voeltz, L. M., and I. M. Evans. 1982. The assessment of behavioral interrelationships in child behavior therapy. *Behavioral Assessment* 4: 131–65.

Wahler, R. G. 1969. Oppositional children: A quest for parental reinforcement control. *Journal of Applied Behavior Analysis* 2: 159–70.

Wahler, R. G. 1975. Some structural aspects of deviant child behavior. *Journal of Applied Behavior Analysis* 8: 27:42.

Wahler, R. G. 1980. The insular mother: Her problems in parent-child treatment. *Journal of Applied Behavior Analysis* 13: 207–19.

Wahler, R. G., and A. D. Afton. 1980. Attentional processes in insular and noninsular mothers. *Child Behavior Therapy* 2: 25–41.

Wahler, R. G., and W. H. Cormier. 1970. The ecological interview: A first step in outpatient child behavior therapy. *Journal of Behavior and Experimental Psychiatry* 1: 279–89.

Wahler, R. G., and J. E. Dumas. 1985. Stimulus class determinants of mother-child coercive interchanges in multidistressed families. In J. Burchard and S. Burchard, eds., *Prevention of Delinquent Behavior.* New York: Sage.

Wahler, R. G., and J. J. Fox. 1980. Solitary toy play and time-out: A family treatment package for children with aggressive and oppositional behavior. *Journal of Applied Behavior Analysis* 13: 23–39.

Wahler, R. G., and J. J. Fox. 1981. Setting events in applied behavior analysis: Toward a conceptual and methodological expansion. *Journal of Applied Behavior Analysis* 14: 327–38.

Wahler, R. G., and M. G. Graves. 1983. Setting events in social networks: Ally or enemy in child behavior therapy? *Behavior Therapy* 14 (1): 19–36.

Wahler, R. G., and D. M. Hann. 1986. The communication patterns of troubled mothers: In search of a keystone in the generalization skills. *Education and Treatment of Children* 26:199–210.

Wahler, R., L. Sansbury, I. Bender, and S. Bryant. 1985, November. Discriminative restructuring of the insular mother's ecosystem. Paper presented at Association for the Advancement of Behavior Therapy, Houston, Texas.

Webster, N. 1975. *Webster's New Twentieth Century Dictionary of the English Language.* New York: World Publishing Company.

Webster-Stratton, C. 1985. Predictors of treatment outcome in parent training for conduct-disordered children. *Behavior Therapy* 16: 223–43.

Wells, K. C. 1981. Assessment of children in outpatient settings. In M. Herson and A. S. Bellack (Eds.), *Behavioral assessment: A practical handbook.* New York: Pergamon Press.

Willems, E. P. 1974. Behavioral technology and behavioral ecology. *Journal of Applied Behavior Analysis* 7: 151–66.

6

Toward an Interbehavioral Medicine

F. Dudley McGlynn, Edwin W. Cook III, and Paul E. Greenbaum

In this chapter we present an interbehavioral view of the activities that fall under the rubric of "behavioral medicine." The chapter begins with an overview of the behavioral medicine movement and a brief history of how and "why" it evolved. The second section of the chapter argues that continuing dialogue about the conceptual organization of behavioral medicine activities is desirable. It then overviews alternative means of conceptual organization and outlines, in more detail, an interbehavioral construction of behavioral medicine. In the third section an ongoing study of mothers and children as they interact in medical settings is described in some detail. It is used to illustrate concretely a methodology that gives expression to interbehavioral postulates. The fourth section is a summary and resume of an interbehavioral medicine. While our focus is behavioral medicine *research*, the chapter can, by implication, serve to alert behavioral medicine practitioners to the benefits of an interbehavioral perspective.

History and Current Status

The behavioral-medicine movement exploded onto the psychological scene at the end of the 1970s. As of the mid–1980s, its participants are engaged in a massive research and clinical effort in which behavioral science principles are brought to bear in understanding, treating, managing, and preventing large numbers of so-called medical problems. Some behavioral-medicine specialists work in already well established research and practice areas—for example, smoking,

The participation of Drs. Cook and Greenbaum was supported by grant #5 T32 DE07133–03 from the National Institute of Dental Research to Dr. Barbara G. Melamed.

obesity, hypertension, headache, asthma, chronic pain, coronary-prone behavior, peripheral vascular disease, and diabetes. Others are carving out new arenas for research and practice—for example, cancer, arthritis, musculoskeletal disorders, and gastrointestinal disorders. (For reviews see *British Journal of Clinical Psycholoy*, vol. 21, pt. 4; *Journal of Consulting and Clinical Psychology*, vol. 50, no. 6; *Journal of Psychosomatic Research*, vol. 26, no. 5.)

O. F. Pomerleau (1982) has described how behavioral medicine evolved. In 1973, the term behavioral medicine was first used in the book *Biofeedback: Behavioral Medicine* (Birk, 1973). In 1974, the Center for Behavioral Medicine was formed at the University of Pennsylvania. Around the same time, the Laboratory for the Study of Behavioral Medicine was formed at Stanford University. In 1977, the Yale Conference on Behavioral Medicine convened the various early participants and produced the first working definition for the new field (Schwartz & Weiss, 1978). The late 1970s and early 1980s witnessed the establishment of various special-interest organizations, such as the Society of Behavioral Medicine, the Academy of Behavioral Medicine Research, and the Division of Health Psychology within the American Psychological Association. Three new journals also were launched during this period: *Health Psychology*, the *Journal of Behavioral Medicine*, and *Behavioral Medicine Abstracts*. Finally, the late 1970s and early 1980s saw the establishment of behavior-medicine funding units within several agencies, for example, the National Cancer Institute; the National Heart, Lung, and Blood Institute; and the National Institute of Dental Research.

E. B. Blanchard (1982) and W. S. Agras (1982) have offered accounts of why behavioral medicine evolved. Blanchard traces its origins to the successes of operant technology with health-related problems such as smoking, to the successes of biofeedback technology with problems such as headache, and to the concurrent recognition in medical and public health circles that *potentially modifiable behaviors* were playing important roles in many serious diseases. Agras (1982) adds that the development of behavioral medicine was fostered by interest in a preventive approach to reducing runaway health-care costs. In any case, there is a new and vigorously developing scientific and professional movement that incorporates research and clinical disciplines that heretofore were not well connected—for example, various behavioral sciences, biomedical sciences, and medical specialties (Agras, 1982). There has been dialogue concerning how such diverse disciplines and activities are to be organized conceptually.

Toward an Interbehavioral Medicine

The practice of behavioral medicine currently is more technological than scientific. In part, this reflects the technological character of behavior modification and biofeedback movements out of which behavioral medicine evolved. Demonstrably effective behavior-change technologies are critical to the survival of behavioral medicine and should constitute the single most important contemporary goal of workers in the field (Agras, 1982). At the same time, some authorities have pointed to the need for a unifying conceptual framework. Some options for the conceptual organization of behavioral medicine are overviewed here by way of setting the stage for an interbehavioral construction of the field.

Classical Behavior Modification

Pomerleau has insisted that the behavior modification tradition should guide the growth of behavioral medicine. "Behavioral medicine can be defined as . . . the clinical use of techniques derived from the experimental analysis of behavior—behavior therapy and behavior modification—for the evaluation, prevention, management, and treatment of physical disease or physiological dysfunction" (Pomerleau & Brady, 1979, p. xiii). Allegiance to the behavior modification movement would have mixed effects on the evolution of behavioral medicine. On the positive side, behavior modification brings with it a history of relatively careful intervention-oriented research and some impressive achievements at the level of behavioral technology. On the negative side, classical behavior modification is too diverse conceptually to foster conceptual order. The theories of Pavlov, Thorndike, Tolman, Guthrie, Skinner, Hull, Mowrer, Wolpe, Sherrington, and Watson have all been influential. Further, the systematic and methodological postures embedded in the origins of classical behavior therapy are oftentimes contradictory. Finally, allegiance to classical behavior therapy and behavior modification will not protect behavioral medicine from mentalistic formulations. Behavior therapy itself has been robbed of its hoped-for behaviorism by reformulations that seem to take the general form of a Hellenistic dualism (e.g., Meichenbaum, 1974).

The Experimental Analysis of Behavior

Several benefits would follow from restricting behavioral medicine activities to those consonant with the experimental analysis of behavior. The three-term contingency (antecedent-behavior-consequence) lends itself readily to behavioral medicine problems such as adherence to prescribed health-care regimes (e.g., Claerhout & Lutzker, 1981) and pain behavior (e.g., Fordyce, 1976). Orthodox behavior analysis methodology focuses attention on individual subjects and on behaviors that are clinically significant. Contemporary treatments of the reinforcement concept (e.g., Baum, 1973) and of environmental settings (e.g., Moxley, 1982) show that behavior analysis is not inherently incompatible with interbehavioral thinking. Hence, continued development of behavioral medicine under the aegis of behavior analysis is to be desired. However, behavior analysis is not without potential shortcomings as a sole organizing schema for behavioral-medicine activities. For example, it does little by way of organizing the diverse biomedical and behavioral-science concepts of which behavioral medicine is comprised.

Systems Theory

Systems theory was developed by interdisciplinary scholars such as W. R. Ashby (1958), L. von Bertalanffy (1950), and J. G. Miller (1978). The twofold goal of systems theory is to promote a unified science by describing common-alities in events across different levels of scientific discourse and to discover *emergent* behaviors of systems in general. G. E. Schwartz (e.g., 1980) has proposed that systems theory provides a conceptual framework for integrating the diverse disciplines involved in behavioral medicine. The proposal holds for connecting established disciplines such as sociology, anthropology, ecology, psychology, ethology, organ physiology, cellular biology, and biochemistry. It holds also for articulating new interdisciplines such as sociobiology, behavioral neuroscience, and psychoneuroendocrinology.

Schwartz's proposal has a good deal of merit. "Living systems" theory (Miller, 1978), for example, describes nineteen common subsystems present in cells, organs, organisms, groups, organizations, societies, and supranational systems. Cybernetic control theory (Weiner, 1948), for another example, is a subset of general systems theory that provides concepts such as negative feedback and homeostasis that can be applied to virtually all scientific disciplines. Delin-eating such commonalities can facilitate the attempts of behavioral-medicine researchers to translate information across interdisciplinary language levels. As with other potential superstructures for behavioral medicine, however, systems theory is not without potential shortcomings. For example, effective use of systems concepts requires familiarity with sciences immediately "above" and "below" the language level of the researcher's basic discipline. In addition, systems thinking does not protect behavioral medicine from mentalistic doctrines. "A sense of hope may be derived from the . . . health system (organization) or family (group), translated into a belief (organism), which acts by way of the cortex . . . to regulate the immune system" (Schwartz, 1980, p. 27).

Interbehavioral Field Theory

A. Einstein and L. Infeld (1938) among others described a three-stage pro-gression in the evolution of physical science thinking. In the first stage, the actions of objects were explained with reference to properties or characteristics *within* the objects. In the second, the actions of objects were explained by reference to causal forces acting *between* objects; the objects themselves being more or less inert mimes of causal mechanics. In the third stage, the actions of objects are construed as participating in concert with the actions of other objects to form continuous natural-event fields. In the case of electromagnetic phenom-ena, for example, "it is not the charges nor the particles, but the field in the space between the charges and the particles which is essential for the description of physical phenomena" (Einstein & Infeld, 1938).

J. R. Kantor shared the three-stage view of the evolution of physical science and set about, early on, to develop interbehavioral field theory as a natural science framework for psychology. The following quotations concerning the field concept and mechanistic causality illustrate Kantor's interbehavioral perspective.

On the field concept for psychology:

For a science such as psychology it is advisable to look upon the field as the entire system of things and conditions operating in any event taken in its available totality. It is only the entire system of factors which will provide proper descriptive and explanatory materials for the handling of events. It is not the reacting organism alone but also the stimulating things and conditions, as well as the setting factors. (Kantor, 1969, pp. 370–71)

On mechanistic causality:

The alternative to the causal construction is the *interbehavioral field*. All creative agencies, all powers and forces are rejected. An event is regarded as a field of factors all of which are equally necessary or, more properly speaking, equal participants in the event. . . . [E]vents are scientifically described by analyzing these participating factors and finding how they are related. (Kantor, 1959, p. 90)

For forty or so years Kantor's integrated field theory prompted virtually no research. During the past decade, however, interbehavioral work has appeared at several places in the literature. Roger D. Ray and his colleagues (e.g., Ray & Brown, 1975) have shown, for animal behavior, that concepts such as reinforcement and learning can be replaced by fine-grained descriptions of momentary configurations involving spatial, temporal, organismic, and historical variables. At a closely related level is work on concurrent (e.g. Henton & Iverson, 1978) and sequential (e.g., Ray, Upson, & Henderson, 1977) "response patterns," wherein it is postulated that behavior is a continuous aggregate flow and is not comprised of discrete events. At a third level is the work of ecological and interbehavioral family-systems therapy researchers (e.g., Wahler & Fox, 1981), wherein field factors such as environmental features and prior interbehavioral field events have been shown to influence rates of aversive mother-child exchanges.

W. H. Redd and F. R. Rusch (1985) used R. A. Moxley's (1982) construction of behaviorally regnant environmental factors in conceptualizing and changing pain/distress behavior among cancer patients. In brief, "enduring setting events" (e.g., the nurse's call button) and "temporary ongoing activity events" (e.g., visitors, laboratory procedures) were shown to relate functionally to the patients' distress behaviors. Hence, thinking that is compatible with Kantor's view of environmental participation in interbehavioral event fields has found its way into the behavioral-medicine literature.

Postulates of an Interbehavioral Medicine

D. J. Delprato and F. D. McGlynn (1986) suggested that Kantor's interbehavioral perspective can serve to organize behavioral-medicine activities and

offered six "postulates for behavioral medicine." In order to set the stage for
discussing research on mother-child interaction in medical settings, the postulates
are summarized here. (a) The events of interbehavioral medicine occur within
integrated multifactor fields that are comprised *solely* of the patient's interactions
with objects, events, and other organisms; the setting factors; and the media of
contact (e.g., light, air) that make the interactions possible. (b) The integrated
multifactor fields are *continuously* evolving so long as the patient is alive. (c)
The entire organism, not only specific components, participates in interbehavior.
(d) An interbehavioral medicine demands cooperation among the various disciplines with specialized knowledge of the participating factors. (e) Clinical and
research procedures in interbehavioral medicine are construed as modifications
of field factors and, hence, of entire interbehavioral fields. (f) The goals of
interventions are alterations in field trajectories, away from disease toward health
and well-being.

Child—Mother Interbehavior in a Medical Setting

Children often display distress in medical settings. These displays interfere
with treatment and with subsequent receipt of health care. Hence, researchers
have sought to identify the causes of such distress, with an eye to reducing or
eliminating it. Not surprisingly, the role of the mother has been the focus of
several investigations. In this section of the chapter we describe our research on
child-mother interactions in medical settings in order to illustrate an evolving
data-analytic approach that gives expression to interbehavioral postulates.

Overview and Critique of Existing Research

Research on maternal influence over children's medical distress has typically
used the mother's presence as a binary variable. Some studies have shown
maternal presence to be associated with increased child distress (e.g., Gross,
Stern, Levin, Dale, & Wojnilower, 1983). Other studies have shown maternal
presence to be associated with decreased child distress (e.g., Hannallah & Rosales, 1983). Still others have shown maternal presence or absence to have no
influence (Venham, 1979). From an interbehavioral-field perspective this empirical confusion is not surprising for at least two reasons. First, binary manipulations of maternal presence versus absence do not specify what the mothers
are *doing* while they are present. Depending, in part, on the type of maternal
behavior, increased, decreased, or unaltered child distress behaviors might be
predicted. Second, even descriptions of how a mother's actions influence her
child's distress behavior would tell only part of the interbehavioral story; for
example, they would not specify how the child's behaviors influence reciprocally
those of the mother or how setting factors contribute to interbehavioral flows.

Some Interbehaviorally Oriented Research

The work to be described here is just one step toward a bona fide interbehavioral research program. It does not deal with "the entire system of things and conditions" that operate when mothers and children interact in medical settings. It does, however, attempt to capture the reciprocal flow of child-mother interbehavior in a way that is highly congruent with field-theoretical thinking.

Research setting and data collection. The primary purpose of the research is to describe the interactive behavior of mothers and children waiting for a pediatric examination. A secondary purpose is to describe differences in mother-child interaction which covary with other variables such as medically related fears, state and trait anxiety. The ultimate goal is the identification of dyads at risk for showing medically related anxiety behaviors that might interfere with optimal treatment and/or with future health-care seeking.

Subjects for this example were forty mother-child dyads awaiting treatment in the outpatient clinic of Shands Teaching Hospital, a tertiary care medical center affiliated with the University of Florida. Dyads with children suffering from chronic or life-threatening diseases were excluded from the sample. After administration of questionnaires, and prior to the arrival of the physician, dyads were videotaped for five to ten minutes in the examination room.

The general approach and basic concepts. The first decision in setting about to characterize a person-person interbehavioral system concerns the initial units of measurement. According to interbehavioral thinking, the behavior life of an organism is absolutely continuous as long as the individual is alive. At one level this conception is problematic since the scientific study of behavior requires discrete observational units. At another level, however, it is not problematic. The "absolutely continuous" nature of behavior simply means that the choice of *any* discrete unit of scientific analysis is somewhat artificial. The seven analytical units used initially in the work described here were maternal reassuring, distracting, informing, ignoring, and agitation, along with child distress and child attachment. The seven variables are construed, a priori, as likely participants in two-behavior interbehavioral systems. As a result of observation and analysis, one or more variables can be described as not participating in a known interbehavioral system. Also as a result of observation and analysis, the two-behavior systems studied initially can be elaborated, ultimately, into N-behavior systems. These variables originated in the literature on mother-child interaction in approach-to-stranger situations (Ainsworth & Wittig, 1969) and preparation for surgery (Melamed, Robbins, & Fernandez, 1982). In addition, L. A. Abeles (1984) and J. P. Bush, B. G. Melamed, P. Sheras, and P. E. Greenbaum (1986) used these behavioral categories in research on mother-child dyads awaiting pediatric examinations. In fact, the present research entails a reanalysis of data produced by these investigators.

A related decision concerns the frequency with which to sample the chosen behaviors. In our work each variable is measured every five seconds, a sampling interval that is presumed to provide sufficient resolution in time to detect temporal relationships among fluctuations.

Another decision is to choose a mathematical approach to describing the system within which pairs of retained variables are participants. Once the system has been tentatively described, a model is developed from which changes in some variables are predicted given changes in others. We use the well-known and flexible General Linear Model (which is implicit in analysis of variance, regression, and correlation) to construct models. The null hypothesis is, at every stage, that there is no temporal relationship between the two behaviors; that is, the variables are so loosely linked as to prompt the conclusion that they are not part of an interbehavioral system. The alternative hypothesis is that behaviors covary *systematically*, and the purpose of the data analysis is to delineate the pattern of covariation and, ultimately, to understand the operating rules of the system.

Only recently have methods been developed that precisely identify sequential patterns in the stream of behavior that occur when two people interact (Budescu, 1984; Cook & Greenbaum, 1987; Gottman, 1979). Three types of sequential patterns are fundamental to the methodological approach: autodependence, cross-dependence, and dominance. *Autodependence* describes how the presence or absence of a behavior at one time point influences the probablility of the same behavior at an adjacent time point. In the abstract, the magnitude of the auto-dependence effect is a function of the duration of a behavior relative to the length of the sampling interval. Whenever a sampling interval is used that ensures high resolution of the behavioral stream, strong autodependence effects are expected. In fact, the absence of a strong autodependence effect is an indication that the sampling frequency is inadequate (Gottman, 1980). Hence, autodependence effects are ubiquitous and large in magnitude when the behavioral stream is sampled adequately, and autodependence should be assessed whenever other factors influencing the probabilities of behaviors are to be evaluated. For the behavioral categories and sampling intervals used here, the autodependence, or "behavioral inertia," effect is quite large in magnitude. If one of the behaviors is occurring, the probability is high that it will still be occurring five seconds later. Likewise, if a behavior is not occurring, its probability of occurrence at the next sampling point is relatively low.

Cross-dependence describes how the presence or absence of a behavior at one point in time influences the probability of a different behavior at an adjacent point in time. The cross-dependence of behavior *A* on behavior *B* refers to the degree to which the presence or absence of behavior *A* is predictable from the immediately prior presence or absence of behavior *B*. Cross-dependence is more complex than autodependence, since two behaviors are involved, and there are two directions for cross-dependence. For example, the cross-dependence of maternal agitation on child distress refers to the predictability of agitation from prior distress, while the cross-dependence of distress on agitation refers to the predictability of distress from prior agitation. Each of these cross-dependencies is examined, and the pattern of relationships between them is used in delineating sequences. If two behaviors covary over time, with neither behavior leading or following the other differentially, and if both behaviors have durations greater than the sampling interval, then the presence or absence of either is equally predictable from the other at the *prior* time point; that is, each behavior is equally cross-dependent on the other.

Dominance (Gottman, 1980) refers to a relationship of unequal cross-dependence. Two behaviors covary but one behavior does consistently occur first. For example, if a mother withholds her reassurance until the child displays distress, then prior distress will predict reassurance more than prior reassurance will predict distress. By testing for dominance relationships within the stream of behavior, we can identify sequences. Thus, dominance provides a basic tool for mapping the temporal order of events in interbehavior. While we cannot conclude with certainty that the dominant behavior paces the other (since both behaviors are imbedded in integrated systems along with other variables), the demonstration of dominance provides the strongest support for this conclusion that is available without an experimental manipulation.

In summary, the concepts of cross-dependence and dominance describe the relationship between two behaviors within an interbehavioral system, while the concept of autodependence makes possible the factoring out of inertia within each behavior. By describing the sequential relationships between all possible pairs of behaviors in these terms we can, ultimately, construct a model of how the N-behavior system performs in the aggregate.

Analysis of a Two-Behavior System: Maternal Agitation and Child Distress. As noted, the characterization of mother-child dyadic interaction is the central focus of the research and an additional interest is describing how the mother-child interaction varies as a function of other field factors. Maternal anxiety in the medical setting possibly is communicated to the child and might be an important field influence on the child's distress or disruptive behavior. In the present example, therefore, we measured how the autodependence, cross-dependence, and dominance relationships within mother-child dyads differed as a function of maternal self-report on a state-anxiety measure (Spielberger, Gorsuch, & Lushene, 1970).

The research currently is restricted to describing the temporal patterning of different pairs of behaviors. In this example we consider mainly one pair (maternal agitation and child distress) in order to present the data analytic process in detail. Questions to be answered are: Is the probability of child distress greater when maternal agitation is present than when agitation is not present? Is child distress more likely to be initiated (i.e., to change from OFF to ON) when maternal agitation is present than when it is not present? Does the pattern of influence between maternal agitation and child distress vary with the mother's report of state anxiety?

We begin by determining interrater reliabilities for the behavior categories used. For the data described here, interrater correlations ranged from .82 to .97. We then calculate eight conditional probabilities for each dyad (see Table 6.1).

Table 6.1
Design for Agitation and Distress Analysis

		Sequence	
Dependent behavior at time $t-1$	Independent behavior at time $t-1$	Predicting Distress from Agitation	Predicting Agitation from Distress
Present	Present	p (D | D ∧ A)	p (A | A ∧ D)
Present	Absent	p (D | D ∧ -A)	p (A | A ∧ -D)
Absent	Present	p (D | -D ∧ A)	p (A | -A ∧ D)
Absent	Absent	p (D | -D ∧ -A)	p (D | -A ∧ -D)

Note. D = distress; A = agitation; - = "not" or "absent"; | = given;

∧ = logical "and."

These probabilities represent the crossing of three factors: sequence, autodependence, and cross-dependence. Sequence refers to the temporal ordering of the two variables; that is, for half of the probabilities (left column in Table 6.1) distress at time t is the dependent variable. For the other half (right column) agitation at time t is the dependent variable. Autodependence refers to whether the behavior we are predicting at time t is present (top two rows) or absent (bottom two rows) at the prior sample point $(t-1)$. Where we are predicting either child distress or maternal agitation at time t, cross-dependence refers to whether the other behavior was present (rows 1 and 3) or absent (rows 2 and 4) at the prior sample point $(t-1)$.

If raw conditional probabilities were used, the expected cell means generated in the analysis could fall outside the range of legitimate probability values (i.e., zero to one). Hence, in the next phase of the analysis, the conditional probabilities are subjected to a logit transformation which is continuous from minus to plus infinity (see Cox, 1970). In addition, the logits of the conditional probabilities are standardized so as to form a uniform scale for comparing different behaviors.

Once the standardized logits of the conditional probabilities are available, the variables of sequence, autodependence, and cross-dependence are represented as within-dyad main effects in an analysis of variance and are combined with the between-dyad main effects for self-reported maternal anxiety. The analysis also yields various interactions. The important concept of dominance, or directionality of influence, is represented in the cross-dependence × sequence interaction. That is, dominance exists when the cross-dependence for one sequence is significantly different from the cross-dependence for the other.

Results of the analysis of variance confirmed the expected large-magnitude autodependence effect, $F(1,18) = 190.8$, $p < .001$. In addition, a significant cross-dependence main effect, $F(1,18) = 12.7$, $p < .01$, and a marginally significant sequence × cross-dependence × maternal anxiety interaction, $F(1,18) = 4.0$, $p < .07$, suggested that sequential relationships between the two variables were present. The significant effects within the omnibus analysis prompted subsequent t-test comparisons of the logits of conditional probabilities for each behavior when the other behavior was previously present and previously absent. These two comparisons were performed for each level of the autodependence factor (same behavior present versus absent during the preceding time interval) and for each level of maternally self-reported state anxiety (high versus low).

Table 6.2 presents these conditional probabilities along with the comparison t-tests. As shown, the dominance relationship between maternal agitation and child distress depended upon the mother's self-report of state anxiety. For dyads with high anxious mothers, maternal agitation was followed by significantly increased child distress, suggesting that maternal agitation was pacing child distress in these dyads. For dyads with low anxious mothers, maternal agitation had no effect on child distress. Child distress, however, was followed by significantly increased maternal agitation. In brief, maternal agitation among high anxious mothers was a precipitant of child distress, while maternal agitation among low anxious mothers was a consequence of child distress.

Toward an N-behavior system. The above analysis was shown in detail for illustrative purposes. Similar data analyses involving two-behavior systems and interacting field factors currently are under way. For example, a similar analysis was applied to the variables of maternal agitation and child attachment. Among dyads with low anxious mothers, agitation was followed by decreased attachment, while in dyads with high anxious mothers, agitation and attachment were not significantly related. The cumulative results of the agitation-distress and agitation-attachment analyses point to two different patterns of mother-child interbehavior. In dyads with high anxious mothers, maternal agitation is a field factor pacing child distress. In dyads with low anxious mothers, child distress is a field factor pacing maternal agitation and the agitation paces attachment.

At the present time the analytic approach limits us to analyzing the pair-wise interrelationships. We have adopted a pragmatic assumption that by cataloguing the two-behavior systems we can, to some degree, understand how the larger system operates. However, the analytic method must be extended to handle N behavioral variables if we are to understand the aggregate interbehavioral flow. This necessity stems from the basic theoretical postulate that interbehavioral fields are integrated, evolving wholes. Thus, the cross-dependence relationship

Table 6.2
Conditional Probabilities of Maternal Agitation and Child Distress

State Anxiety	Distress Effects on Agitation			Agitation Effects on Distress		
	Agit|–Dtrs	Agit|Dtrs	t	Dtrs|–Agit	Dtrs|Agit	t
High (N = 8)	.39	.43	(1.34)	.51	.61	(2.27)*
Low (N = 12)	.37	.43	(2.81)*	.49	.46	(–0.60)

Note. Agit = Agitation; Dtrs = Distress, | = given; – = "not" or
        "absent."

* p < .05.

between behavior A and behavior B is presumed to depend on whether behavior C is present or absent. In order to incorporate this presumption, the within-dyad design matrix shown in Table 6.1 would need to be doubled, such that half of the resulting set of probabilitites were conditional upon C being present, and the other half upon C being absent. However, C also is presumed to be cross-dependent in relationship to A and B. A complete analysis would delineate these relationships as well. Ultimately, multivariate statistics will be used in describing the flows of N-behavior systems. We are only beginning such an analytic approach. The difficulties in constructing statistical models of the "entire system of things and conditions" are real (Rosenfeld & Remmers, 1981), but statistical approaches to problems that are similar to ours have been developed (e.g., Porges, Bohrer, Cheung, Drasgow, McCabe, & Keren, 1980).

Summary and Resume of Interbehavioral Medicine

Behavioral medicine is a recent development on the psychological scene. It has origins in behavior modification and biofeedback and entails diverse applications of behavioral-science principles to so-called medical problems. It is a vigorous and growing movement complete with journals, professional societies, funding agencies, and so forth. Classical behavior modification, experimental analysis of behavior, and systems theory have all been proposed as organizing schema for the field. This chapter proposed that Kantor's interbehavioral field theory also can serve as an organizing schema. It reiterated some postulates for an "interbehavioral medicine" and showed the beginning stages of research on mother-child interaction in medical settings that are highly congruent with interbehavioral theory.

We have not argued here that interbehavioral field theory should immediately replace behavior modification, behavior analysis, or even systems theory as *the* organizing schema for behavioral medicine. As our own research shows, a great deal of work remains before an interbehavioral medicine can become a reality. Even so, the resume of an interbehavioral approach is summarized in closing.

Behavior modification is technologically satisfactory, but it suffers from methodological pluralism and has drifted into a Hellenistic mind-body position. The interbehavioral alternative can incorporate the technologies, while homogenizing methodological approaches and guarding against spiritualistic mind-body positions. Behavior analysis is technologically satisfactory and methodologically cohesive. However, it has been insufficiently concerned with the complexity of both organismic and environmental setting conditions and it has been excessively concerned with the unidirectional control of organisms by environments. The interbehavioral alternative again can incorporate the technology while explicitly redressing these errors of focus. Systems theory can serve as a source of new concepts and as an aid to interdisciplinary communication. However, unrestrained systems theory is clearly vulnerable to mentalistic doctrines. The interbehavioral alternative can take advantage of systems science (i.e., mathematics) while maintaining the natural science perspective that is the essence of behaviorism.

References

Abeles, L. A. 1984. Mother-child interaction in a medical setting: Attachment effects on distress. Unpublished master's thesis, University of Florida.

Agras, W. S. 1982. Behavioral medicine in the 1980s: Nonrandom connections. *Journal of Consulting and Clinical Psychology* 50: 797–803.

Ainsworth, M.D.S., and B. A. Wittig. 1969. Attachment and exploratory behavior of one year olds in a strange situation. In B. M. Foss (Ed.), *Determinants of infant behavior*, vol. 4. London: Methuen.

Ashby, W. R. 1958. General systems theory as a new discipline. In L. von Bertalanffy and A. Rapoport (Eds.), *General systems: Yearbook of the Society for General Systems Research* 3:1–6.

Baum, W. M. 1973. The correlation-based law of effect. *Journal of the Experimental Analysis of Behavior* 20:137–53.

Bertalanffy, L. von 1950. An outline of general systems theory. *British Journal of the Philosophy of Science* 1:134–64.

Birk, L. 1973. *Biofeedback: Behavioral medicine*. New York: Grune & Stratton.

Blanchard, E. B. 1982. Behavioral medicine: Past, present, and future. *Journal of Consulting and Clinical Psychology* 50:795–96.

Budescu, D. V. 1984. Tests of lagged dominance in sequential dyadic interaction. *Psychological Bulletin* 96:402–14.

Bush, J. P., B. G. Melamed, P. Sheras, and P. E. Greenbaum. 1986. Mother-child patterns of coping with anticipatory medical stress. *Health Psychology* 5:137–57.

Claerhout, S., and J. R. Lutzker. 1981. Increasing children's self-initiated compliance to dental regimens. *Behavior Therapy* 12:383–99.

Cook, E. W., III, and P. E. Greenbaum. 1987. Least squares sequential analysis: Untangling patterns of cross-dependence and dominance. Submitted for publication.

Cox, D. R. 1970. *The analysis of binary data*. London: Methuen.

Delprato, D. J., and F. D. McGlynn. 1986. Innovations in behavioral medicine. In M. Hersen, R. M. Eisler, and P. M. Miller (Eds.), *Progress in behavior modification*. New York: Academic Press.

Einstein, A., and L. Infeld. 1938. *The evolution of physics*. New York: Simon & Schuster.

Fordyce, W. E. 1976. *Behavior methods for chronic pain and illness*. St. Louis: Mosby.

Gottman, J. M. 1979. Time-series analysis of continuous data in dyads. In M. E. Lamb, S. J. Suomi, and G. R. Stephenson (Eds.), *Social interaction analysis: Methodological issues*. Madison: University of Wisconsin Press.

Gottman, J. M. 1980. Analysis for sequential connection and assessing interobserver reliability for the sequential analysis of observational data. *Behavioral Assessment* 2:361–68.

Gross, A. M., R. M. Stern, R. B. Levin, J. Dale, and D. A.Wojnilower. 1983. The effect of mother-child separation on the behavior of children experiencing a diagnostic medical procedure. *Journal of Consulting and Clinical Psychology* 51:783–85.

Hannallah, R. S., and J. K. Rosales. 1983. Experience with parents' presence during anesthesia induction in children. *Canadian Anesthesiology Society Journal* 30: 286–89.

Henton, W. W., and I. H. Iverson. *Classical conditioning and operant conditioning: A response pattern analysis*. New York: Springer-Verlag.

Kantor, J. R. 1959. *Interbehavioral psychology*. Granville, Ohio: Principia Press.

Kantor, J. R. 1969. *The scientific evolution of psychology*, vol. 2. Chicago: Principia Press.

Meichenbaum, D. H. 1974. *Cognitive behavior modification*. Morristown, N.J.: General Learning Press.

Melamed, B. G., R. L. Robbins, and J. Fernandez. 1982. Factors to be considered in psychological preparation for surgery. In D. Routh and M. Wolraich (Eds.), *Advances in developmental and behavioral pediatrics*, vol. 3. New York: JAI Press.

Miller, J. G. 1978. *Living systems*. New York: McGraw-Hill.

Moxley, R. A. 1982. Graphics for three-term contingencies. *The Behavior Analyst*, 5: 45–51.

Pomerleau, O. F. 1982. A discourse on behavioral medicine: Current status and future trends. *Journal of Consulting and Clinical Psychology* 50:1030–39.

Pomerleau, O. F., and J. P. Brady. 1979. *Behavioral medicine: Theory and practice*. Baltimore: Williams & Wilkins.

Porges, S. W., R. E. Bohrer, M. N. Cheung, F. Drasgow, P. McCabe, and G. Keren. 1980. New time-series statistics for detecting rhythmic co-occurrence in the frequency domain: The weighted coherence and its application to psychophysiological research. *Psychological Bullitin* 88:580–87.

Ray, R. D., and Brown, D. A. 1975. A systems approach to behavior. *Psychological Record* 25:459–478.

Ray, R. D., J. D. Upson, and B. J. Henderson. 1977. A systems approach to behavior III: Organismic pace and complexity in time-space fields. *Psychological Record* 27:649–82.

Redd, W. H., and F. R. Rusch. 1985. Behavioral analysis in behavioral medicine. *Behavior Modification* 9:131–54.

Rosenfeld, H. M., and W. W. Remmers. 1981. Searching for temporal relationships in mother-infant interactions. In B. Hoffer and R. St. Clair (Eds.), *Developmental kinesics: The emerging paradigm*. Baltimore: University Park Press.

Schwartz, G. E. 1980. Behavioral medicine and systems theory: A new synthesis. *National Forum* 4:25–30.

Schwartz, G. E., and S. M. Weiss. 1978. Yale conference on behavioral medicine: A proposed definition and statement of goals. *Journal of Behavioral Medicine* 1:3–12.

Spielberger, C. D., R. L. Gorsuch, and R. Lushene. 1970. *State-Trait Anxiety Inventory*. Palo Alto, Calif.: Consulting Psychologists Press.

Venham, L. L. 1979. The effect of the mother's presence on the child's response to a stressful situation. *Journal of Dentistry for Children* 46:219–25.

Wahler, R. G., and J. J. Fox. 1981. Setting events in applied behavior analysis: Toward a conceptual and methodological expansion. *Journal of Applied Behavior Analysis* 14: 327–38.

Wiener, N. 1948. *Cybernetics or control and communication in the animal and machine*. Cambridge, Mass.: MIT Press.

7

Q Methodology: Interbehavioral and Quantum Theoretical Connections in Clinical Psychology

William Stephenson

The word "clinical" has the meaning of patients being treated at their bedsides, each an individual case. The present chapter concerns the methodology and psychology of the $n = 1$ situation, the "single case."

The present author has a long interest in clinical psychology, dating from 1927, his first publication having the title "A Case of General Inertia" (Stephenson, 1931). At that time his mentor, Charles Spearman, of factor-theory fame, had developed a methodology for psychometry (R), requiring large populations of *individuals* for its foundations; his assistant, myself, had been trained as a physicist and felt from the beginning of his career in psychology that the statistical logic of Spearman's psychometry should be as applicable to large populations of *feeling* expressed by a "single case" as it was to large populations of individuals in psychometry. Thus, Q methodology was evolved, where $n = 1$ (Brown, 1968; Burt, 1981; cf. Roseboom, 1972).

There is more to this, however, than a transposition of numbers. If there is a "new realism" in psychology, a new paradigm in its philosophy of science, in which rules of evidence, discovery, and explanation are undergoing dramatic change, then Q has been so involved for fifty years. Q methodology is Einsteinian, where the concern is with relativity and unpredictability. It is into this that we are to venture for clinical psychology, where the involvement is with *states of feeling* at fundamental levels (Stephenson, 1982b, 1983).

The Behavioral Segment

The psychological theory, in outline, begins with any *behavioral segment* of a person (Stephenson, 1953a, 1980, 1982a; Kantor, 1959), such as a patient's concern about a headache. The narrative from the patient about this has a beginning and an end, and it can all be reported. The problem is, how do we deal with it? Give aspirin? Or consider the segment and its narrative? In Q methodology we take the latter course. All the self-referent statements that the patient makes about his or her headache, or *could* make (since the patient shares a culture), constitutes a *concourse*. A concourse is a "population" of statements, not a statement of fact.

Consider the first difficulty: what is self-referent? To say "I have a headache" would ordinarily recommend itself as a statement of fact, even though "I" have said it. To say "I have an excruciating headache" could well be more than a statement of fact—the person may be lying, or exaggerating, or calling attention to something other than a headache—and this would be not only self-referent but also emotionally involved. The concern in Q, and in every concourse, is with the latter. Ordinarily, statements of fact are subject to proof or disproof; statements of self-reference with emotional attachments are not. Thus, if the patient has a high temperature and fibrillating pulse, one would accept as true the statement "I have an excruciating headache." You would be doubtful if "excruciating" was not qualified by such medical signs.

Toward a Theory of Self

Our theory of self stems from this course: every behavioral segment has a corresponding concourse of self-referent (emotional) statements. It is in terms of the concourse that we extract, from the patient, what self-references are involved.

In this connection we see self-reference as an active, not a passive, reaction, because a person organizes purpose in life about a consistent self, of intention at least. The individual, in looking back upon behavior once experienced, can represent a thousand different selves—as boy or girl, adolescent, in marriage, in every remembered incident in a life (Jacobson, 1964). Virginia Woolf (1928), in her "autobiographical" novel *Orlando*, tells it well. She looks back and sees there

selves of which we are built up, one on top of another, as plates are piled on a waiter's hand, have attachments elsewhere, sympathies, little constitutions and rights of their own, call them what you will (and for many of these things there is no name) so that one will come only if it is raining, another in a room with green curtains, another when Mrs. Jones is not there, another if you can promise a glass of wine—and so on; for everybody can multiply from his own experience the different terms which his different selves have made with him—and some are too wildly ridiculous to be mentioned in print at all. (p. 200)

How perceptive indeed! Each recall, each a behavioral segment, has its own "attachments," its own "constitution and rights." And for each of even the

apparently trivial remembrances of Virginia Woolf—the room with green curtains, the promise of a glass of wine—our methodology and theory applies. How
much more, then, can we expect from dramatic episodes in life—normal or
abnormal—this is what subjective science is about. In particular, we can now
take a measure of these bountiful selves. The theory is to the effect that "selves"
form in relation to concourse, creatively, *ab initio*.

A Cup of Tea as Lived Experience

It happens that I knew an Englishman who suffered (his wife said) from an
obsession about things pertaining to bone china, tea making, style and manners
in tea serving—to the point of fastidiousness. Asked about making a good cup
of tea, he would reply all subjectively about "my wife thinks I'm nuts about
china"; "tea for breakfast is one thing, but for teatime it is quite something
else"; "a silver tray at teatime is essential"; "the very feel of bone china is
exquisite"; "my Royal Doulton is for special occasions"; "tea making is a
mystery from China." His concern was with subjective matters involving self-
esteem. It was easy to collect a hundred self-referent (emotive) statements from
the English gentleman's narrative, the concourse for the behavioral segment
constituted by his obsessiveness about tea and teacups.

The *theory of concourse* (Stephenson, 1978) asks that we regard the collection
of statements as a statistical population, to which statistical theory can apply
(Stephenson, 1953b; Sunoo, 1967). A Q-sample is drawn; in the present case it
was thirty-six statements with which the patient performed a set of Q-sorts for
the following theoretical frequency distribution of scores:

Q-Sort Distribution

	Positive Feeling				Neutral		Negative Feeling		
Score	+4	+3	+2	+1	0	−1	−2	−3	−4
Frequency	2	3	4	6	6	6	4	3	2 $n = 36$

Most psychologists now know what a Q-sort is. But if anyone does not know,
it consists of the Q-sorter (patient) scoring the Q-sample on the theoretical
distribution (usually called a "forced" distribution). The Q-sample statements
are each on playing cards, which are shuffled like a pack of cards for a game
of poker; they are read through by the Q-sorter and then distributed for *saliency
of feeling*. Two statements felt about most *positively* gain +4, and so on, the
Q-sorter proceeding from one side to the other, leaving six to score zero in the
middle. This is a theoretical requirement and it is widely misunderstood. The
statements have no normative value; they are like equal marbles in a bag and

Table 7.1
"Vital Sign" for the Patient before Treatment

Conditions of Instruction	Operant Factors		
	I	II	III
1. Present feeling (<u>now</u>)	X		
2. Precipitating incident			-X
3. Condition before coming to U.S.A.		X	
4. Connoisseur's feeling	X		
5. Wife's feeling			
6. Typical American's feeling		X	
7. Ideal feeling			
8. What Mother felt			X

<u>Note.</u> X = significant loading, all other values insignificant.

gain their saliency only in the act of Q-sorting. Thus, each statement may have different meanings in different Q-sorts and mean different things to different people. This should be obvious: the baby who says "da-da" expresses quite different meanings when it sees its father unexpectedly, or when it hears him coming from another room, or when he or she cuddles into him in warm embrace—yet "da-da" is the same, except for different emotional emphases. But so it is about every self-referent statement in every concourse; meanings are what the given situation and Q-sort instruction require.

In the present example, before treatment began, the patient performed eight Q-sorts with the Q-sample, spread over two days, with the eight different conditions of instruction given in Table 7.1. The conditions are the scientist's experimental design, to probe into the behavioral segment. The Q-sorts were factor analyzed for the 8 × 8 matrix of correlations, providing factors I, II, III. We shall take the factor analysis for granted; it is possible to follow our argument with only a modicum of knowledge about factor theory. The factors are theoretical Q-sorts, like any empirically performed, as if the mind had performed them, unknown to the patient. They are therefore distinct selves of the patient, such as Virginia Woolf described, attached to a particular event or experience in the patient's life. They can be assessed and shown as Q-sorts to the patient to see if they are recognized as such selves, and they usually are. Clearly, there are only a few of hundreds that could be "called upon," each with its own experiential or fantasy attachments.

In the above case factor I apparently represents the self *now*, as *connoisseur* (Q-sorts 1 and 4 are on the same factor), and this is probably the core representation of the obsessiveness about tea matters. Factor II suggests a *mundane* self, of disparagement or the like. Factor III is also pertinent to the clinical problem, with mother at one extreme (positive) and the precipitating cause (negative) at the other.

One may appreciate why this is called a "vital sign" (Stephenson, 1985). Every behavioral segment, about any behavior, from mention of a headache to reflection upon a volume of autobiographical narrative, from a dream to a delusionary system, can be represented by an operant factor system representing the "selves" at issue. The secret, if any, is in developing the concourse and in designing an appropriate set of conditions of instruction.

Moreover, a "reading" of the "sign" can be taken during the course of treatment or at its conclusion. Or, if one pursues Q methodology as treatment to elicit selves and to enter into discussion about them systematically, the procedure is the same. In the present case a "reading" was taken at completion of psychological treatment. Two additional Q-sorts were performed by the patient, one (Q-sort 1) for his feeling now and another (Q-sort 7) for his ideal now. These, along with the initial Q-sorts 2, 3, 4, 5, 6, and 8 of Table 7.1 were entered into the 8 × 8 matrix, factor analyzed, with the results shown in Table 7.2.

This time there are only two factors, *A* and *B*. It looks as though what was factor III (Table 7.1) has been absorbed by factor *A* (what was factor I), leaving factor II more or less intact, as mundane and perhaps disparaging even of connoisseurs.

Clearly a considerable change has occurred, and we need not ask why for the present purpose. What is important at present is that such "vital signs" are achieved without use of norms; only the patient's subjectivity is at issue. Many years of experimenting have gone into qualifying what data such as these mean. Operant factor structures are natural expressions, independent of the instrumentation in any causative manner (Kantor, 1970). It does not matter what the size is of the Q-sample, or its constitution, or the Q-sort distribution, or the conditions of instruction. Some such operant factor structure will present itself to much the same end in conclusions.

Formalization

As we see, a behavioral segment is the beginning of Q and of subjective (self) science. Each segment is represented by its own concourse of self-referent (emotional, declarative) statements. A Q-sample is taken from the concourse. In reading through its disparate statements the subject is put in touch with the behavioral segment by self-reflection. A Q-sort is an expression of feeling about

Table 7.2
"Vital Sign" for the Patient after Treatment

Conditions of Instruction	Operant Factors	
	A	B
1. Present feeling (<u>now</u>)	X	
2. Precipitating incident	-X	
3. Condition before coming to U.S.A.		X
4. Connoisseur's feeling	X	
5. Wife's feeling		
6. Typical American's feeling		X
7. Ideal feeling	X	
8. What Mother felt	X	

<u>Note</u>. X = significant loading, all other values insignificant.

it, for a given condition of instruction. Unknown to the subject, these conditions can be indicative of the known laws which, though lawful, are not predictive (Popper, 1959; Stephenson, 1978).

The conditions of instruction, however, can also be directly related to the behavioral segment, without assuming these laws. For this we make use of Kantor's (1953) interbehavioral formulation for a psychological event (PE), as follows:

$$PE = C(k, \mathit{sf}, \mathit{rf}, \mathit{hi}, \mathit{st}, \mathit{md}) \tag{1}$$

where C indicates that everything within the parentheses is interactional and subject to scientific inferential behavior; k symbolizes that the segment is unique; and the other symbols stand for stimulus function (sf), response function (rf), historical connections (hi), the immediate setting (st), and the medium of the segment (md). Each of these is defined for us by the patient. Thus, for a patient worried about a headache, sf would be what objects typically brought on the headache, rf would be how the patient behaves during the headache, hi would be past incidents pertinent to both sf and sr, st could be a pressing need to get back to work, and md could be the temperature in the room (intensifying the headache).

This formulation implies a stimulus-response foundation, but it has no such implication for Q, serving only to "set the stage" for probing into the segment. Each of the substantive symbols is represented in Q by one or more Q-sorts, each for a different condition of instruction. The formulation therefore becomes

$$PE = C(k, \text{Q-sort } 1, 2, 3 \ldots) \tag{2}$$

where symbols C, k, are as before. These, duly factor analyzed, provide operant factor structure and factor arrays, to which I shall attend below. It should be said, however, that there never are factors for sf, rf, hi, st, or md; nothing about the expression is predictable in terms of previously stated hypotheses.

In the example for the English gentleman, the eight Q-sorts had reference to expression (1): sf was the purchase of still another expensive tea set which he felt had upset his wife; incidents in the history (hi) were manifest, for example, his mother's fashionable tea parties; the immediate setting (st) was his feeling of wifely unhappiness about his expensive obsession; md was keeping the light bright to see his tea set better; and rf was tension and a gnawing need for treatment. Thus, the conditions of instruction can come from two sources, known laws or direct representation of the segment. Note that the term "psychological event" (PE) remains, but it is only with behavioral (communicable), not physical, implications (cf. Kantor, 1975, 1978).

Factor Arrays

In addition to the factor structures of Tables 7.1 and 7.2 the computer provides two tables in relation to each for their *factor arrays*.

A factor array is a list of the Q-sample statements, each with the score it gained for the factor, in standard statistical terms (quantal units, mean O, standard deviation 1.00, the same unit for all factors). For factor 1 of Table 7.1, the array began with the statement gaining highest positive score, as follows:

I suppose I'm fastidious, but making tea is a ritual for me (score $+1.98$)... and so on, every statement its own score, down to that given largest negative score, viz:

Who on earth, except Americans, would drink tea from a mug? (score -2.07)

Factors are syntheses: each is a theoretical Q-sort, as if performed secretly by the patient. We have to suppose that the synthesis stems from feeling-states, in line with Charles Spearman's theory (1939). Thus, faced with a Q-sort representing a factor, the clinician has to pursue a search for *meaning, by reexperiencing the feelings that could have entered into the synthesis by the unknowing patient*. The clinician has no doubt to draw upon experience and self-knowledge; basically, it is a matter of understanding, of abducing what overall feeling must be involved.

Thus, before treatment, I considered that the feeling-states could be stated, briefly, as *fastidiousness*, *distance*, and *resentment*, respectively, for factors I, II, and III of Table 7.1. Each is a sharp segregation, indicating sharply differentiated selves. It seems that factor I had reference to the patient's overt behavior—meticulous, effeminate, stylish, mannered. Factor II pointed to the disdain and uncivility about those who did not share his fastidiousness. And factor III clearly had reference to annoyance with regard to insinuations about breast-fixation, femininity, and so on. The three were complementary aspects of the behavioral segment; one could not put them together to form another total, feeling-tone. One had to suppose that the factor structure was not "authentic"— that he could have been different, except that the feeling-state behind factor I was likely to be a fixture. In some sense it was more "him" than the feeling-states for factors II and III. Note that aspects of self are fundamentally at issue.

After treatment there was clearly a considerable change. For factors *A* and *B* of Table 7.2 the feeling states were *competency* and *acceptance*, respectively. The patient, in factor *A*, was now able to give realistic advice about how to make a good cup of tea, whereas before treatment he had laced it with his obsession. Factor *B* is evidence that he is no longer fraught with annoyance and resentment at others. Even this self was more "authentic," more accepting of the reality around him.

The change is in line with Perlin's law and also with Parloff's law (Stephenson, 1974). The latter says that we can expect a patient's outward behavior to follow "me" factors. Behavior modification, in short, follows in the wake of "me" more than "mine" factors. In the above case, modification was achieved but also offered some proof by measurement.

Intersubjectivity

There is also the question of intersubjectivity. This is not Popper's criterion for "truth," whereby hypotheses call for intersubjectivite testing (Popper, 1959, p. 46); it is a concern with *subjectivity* (experience) as such (e.g., Koffka, 1935; Kantor, 1959; Maslow, 1966).

In *Psychoanalysis and Q-methodology* (1954) I reported an experiment in which an analyst (*An*) and patient (*Pt*) cooperated to represent each other, with the operant factor structure in Table 7.3. There were ninety-six statements in the Q-sample. The analyst performed three Q-sorts, 1, 2, and 3, for a Q-sample ($n = 96$) of the analytic concourse; *Pt* performed the other four Q-sorts, 4, 5, 6, and 7.

Factor I is limited to *An*.

Factor II is limited to *Pt*.

Factor III joins *An* and *Pt*, and the question arises, is it merely that *An* has correctly *predicted* what *Pt* feels *now* (Q-sort 2 is on factor II), or have *An* and *Pt* experienced intersubjectivity? It is clearly not the latter, because there is no corresponding loading by *Pt* on factor 1 (as is possible for Q-sort 5). (I have

Table 7.3
"Vital Sign" for an Analytic Situation

Conditions of Instruction	Operant Factors		
	I	II	III
1. An: Best Self	X		
2. An: Pt Now		X	
3. An: Now	X		
4. Pt: Before analysis		X	
5. Pt: An now	[ ]		X
6. Pt: Pt. now		X	
7. Pt: Best Self			X

Note. X = significant loading, all others insignificant.

indicated with brackets, [], where the factor loading would be if *Pt* had predicted the analyst's self correctly).

The joining of *An* and *Pt* in the above "vital sign"is because of *An*'s correct prediction of *Pt* by *An*. The analyst appears to be in a transference situation with his patient, perceiving *Pt* as like himself (Q-sort 2 is on factor I, representing *An*). Moreover, according to Rogers' law, *An* is well adjusted (Q-sorts 1 and 3 are on the one factor). The patient is not well adjusted (Q-sorts 6 and 7 are on different factors). But *Pt* is also apparently in a transference situation with the analyst (Q-sort 7 and Q-sort 5 are on the same factor, an idealized *self* having congruence with what *Pt* feels *An* is like now). Could, then, such parallelism in transference be regarded as evidence of intersubjectivity?

Whatever the answer, it should be obvious that there is now a way to ask questions about the possibility of intersubjectivity and this is the way of science. For the present, I prefer to retain the premise that subjectivity is specific to each person. The answer to the question raised by Kohut (1984) as to how analysis brings about a "cure," is answered in Q in terms of processes, as yet little understood, but which involve self-reference and creativity at the covert level of Q methodology, that is, in terms of factors issuing from states of feeling. And how far a "cure" has been achieved must be in relation to two laws to which we have given little attention, Parloff's (that attitudes are in relation to a patient's factors) and Perlin's (that change is in relation to existing "me" factors). All such is commensurable, as "vital sign" measurements.

Conclusion

Our is concern with common speeech. It is indulged, Kantor (1952) once said,

for purposes of play, as a substitute for action, to deceive people, to hide one's thought (Talleyrand), to conceal the fact that one has no thought (Kierkegaard) and for many other purposes. (p. 70)

Amongst the many other purposes is everything subjective in clinical psychology. Concourse is common speech in its subjective mode and, until Newtonian science came along it was the customary mode even among scholars.

By way of Q technique and its methodology we can fathom what a patient is substituting for action, what it is deceptive about, what thoughts are hidden, and indeed whether it has any thought at all. Q-sorting is backward looking (though it can also look forward, especially about intentions), and there are thousands of selves to preview, for anyone, if a scientist is so inclined. The significance of concourse is paramount in this: there is a lexical foundation, but upon this innumerable interbehaviors can be played, no less for a baby and "da-da" than for a Virginia Woolf and *Orlando* or an English gentleman and his tea fetish. Each behavioral segment can have its own "vital sign," each with its own "constitution" and subject to complementarity (as in nuclear physics, where different, even contradictory, aspects can be represented in mathematical space of factor theory). Factor structures are not fixtures made of cardboard; they are slices across active, forward-moving, backward-looking selfhoods. And there are "rights." Some come by laws obeyed by factor structures, except that by laws we mean not merely regularities in nature but also instructions, telling the scientist for what to look.

Q offers a fundamental theory of subjectivity, beginning and ending with expressions of self-reference: we see *selves* in abundance, all about self-reflections upon behavioral segments, minute or long-lasting, and all are self-designing. Amongst them are the episodes of illness to which patients attest. These, however, are not attributes of illness, helplessness, anxiety, depression, anger, humor, competence, or whatever; they are concrete behaviors—it is a cretin boy, in every case, displaying his penis on Hampstead Heath. All current fashions of clinical treatment such as are subjective, from psychoanalytic to hermeneutic, come under Q's sovereignty. The psychoanalytic unconscious is merely Q's factorial space. Hermeneutics remains as a clinician's *understanding* of a case, governed, however, by *factors* in Q's case.

And all remains within the probabilistic framework of quantum theory, where states of feeling, not particulate feelings, are at issue (Zimmerman, 1979). It is the unpredictable electron and unpredictable self, both representable in sciences with common foundations.

References

Atwood, G. E., and R. D. Stolorow. 1984. *Structures of subjectivity: Explorations in psychoanalytic phenomenology*. Hillsdale, N.J.: Analytic Press.

Brown, S. R. 1968. Bibliography on Q technique and its methodology. *Perceptual and Motor Skills*, Monograph Supplement, 4:V26.

Burt, C. 1981. O, P, Q, and R techniques. *Operant Subjectivity* 4:102–19.

Freud, S. 1910. Formulations regarding the two principles in mental functioning. *Collected Papers*, vol. IV. London: Hogarth Press, pp. 13–21.

Jacobson, E. 1964. *The self and the object world*. New York: International Universities Press.

Kantor, J. R. 1952. *An objective psychology of grammar*. Bloomington, Ind.: Principia Press.

Kantor, J. R. 1953. *The logic of modern science*. Bloomington, Ind.: Principia Press.

Kantor, J. R. 1959. *Interbehavioral psychology*. Bloomingon, Ind.: Principia Press.

Kantor, J. R. 1970. An analysis of the experimental analysis of behavior (TEAB). *Journal of the Experimental Analysis of Behavior* 13:101–8.

Kantor, J. R. 1975. Psychology, physics and metaphysics. *Mexican Journal of Behavior Analysis* 1:31–38.

Kantor, J. R. 1978. Cognition as events and as psychic constructions. *Psychological Record* 38:329–42.

Kantor, J. R. 1979. Wundt, experimental psychology and natural science. *Mexican Journal of Behavior Analysis* 5:117–29.

Koffka, K. 1935. *Principles of Gestalt psychology*. London: Kegan, Paul, Trench, & Trubner.

Kohut, H. 1984. *How does analysis cure?* Chicago: University of Chicago Press.

Maslow, A. H. 1966. *The psychology of science*. New York: Harper & Row.

Popper, K. R. 1959. *The logic of scientific discovery*. New York: Basic Books.

Rozeboom, W. W. 1972. Scientific inference: The myth and the reality. In S. R. Brown and D. J. Brenner (Eds.), *Science, psychology and communication: Essays honoring William Stephenson*. New York: Teachers College Press.

Spearman, C. E. 1939. *Psychology down the ages*, vols. I, II. London: Macmillan.

Stephenson, W. 1931. Studies in experimental psychiatry. I. A case of general inertia. *Journal of Mental Science* 78:723–41.

Stephenson, W. 1953a. Postulates of behaviorism. *Philosophy of Science* 20:110–20.

Stephenson, W. 1953b. *The study of behavior: Q-technique and its methodology*. Chicago: University of Chicago Press.

Stephenson, W. 1954. *Psychoanalysis and Q-methodology*. Unpublished manuscript.

Stephenson, W. 1974. Methodology of single case studies. *Journal of Operational Psychiatry* 2:3–16.

Stephenson, W. 1978. Concourse theory of communication. *Communication* 3:21–40.

Stephenson, W. 1980. Consciring: Theory of subjective communicability. *Communication Yearbook 4*. New Brunswick, N.J.: Transaction Books.

Stephenson, W. 1982a. Newton's fifth rule and Q-methodolog𝑦. Application to self-psychology. *Operant Subjectivity* 5 (2):37–57.

Stephenson, W. 1982b. Q-methodology, interbehavioral psychology, and quantum theory. *Psychological Record* 32:235–48.

Stephenson, W. 1983. Quantum theory and Q-methodology: Fictionalistic and probabilistic theories conjoined. *Psychological Record* 33:213–30.

Stephenson, W. 1985. Perspectives in psychology: Integration in clinical psychology. *Psychological Record* 35:41–48.

Sunoo, D. 1967. Q-methodological study of consumer behavior. Unpublished doctoral dissertation, University of Missouri, Columbia.

Woolf, V. 1928. *Orlando: A biography*. New York: Penguin Books.

Zimmerman, D. W. 1979. Quantum theory and interbehavioral psychology. *Psychological Record* 29: 473–85.

8

Assumptions about Teaching Assertiveness: Training the Person or Behavior?

Douglas H. Ruben and Marilyn J. Ruben

The last decade has witnessed an explosion of interest and research on assertiveness behavior and social skills (Ruben, 1985). Assertiveness training is a widely practiced therapy that seeks to resolve interpersonal conflict through the acquisition of effective communication skills. The enormous impact of assertiveness training is largely due to its documented effectiveness in different settings and for a variety of clients (Alberti, 1977; Whitely & Flowers, 1978). Assertiveness programs emphasize direct, confrontive, and dyadic approaches to improving interpersonal adjustment.

Many of today's training programs are offered during regular work or evening hours, systematically spread over a defined period of time. Program objectives and goals deal with coping adjustments, use of disciplinary action, and problem-solving abilities related to personal responsibility. They revolve around three training components: *acquisition, maintenance*, and *follow-up*. Acquisition involves learning the basic model for assertiveness, be it through behavioral or cognitive methods. Behavioral methods stress modeling and rehearsal of realistic or simulated behaviors (e.g., Brown & Brown, 1980; Galassi & Galassi, 1978). Cognitive methods by contrast, aim to alter attitudes and irrational beliefs that are assumed to underlie passivity and aggression (Lange, Rimm, & Loxley, 1975; Rathus, 1975). Maintenance and follow-up simply refer to secondary and tertiary phases of training for the transfer of skills from training setting to those settings conducive to appropriate assertiveness.

The success of this threefold approach is not without serious drawbacks. This chapter first reviews the traditional methodology of assertiveness training and then challenges an assumption of its training philosophy. Specifically, the process of training draws an artificial distinction between the "training" and "real-life" applications. This artificiality derives from the belief that a behavior in one setting will automatically transfer or generalize to another setting through some intrapsychic (personality) dynamic exerting trainees to make this transition. Intrapsychic dynamics such as attitude changes, beliefs, expectations, and feelings, albeit with important referents, contribute minimally to skill generalization or to decisions appropriate for assertive skills. Training programs that make this assumption establish as goals the restructuring of personality, values clarification, and identity awareness. In this respect, consideration is given to changes inside the person rather than to changes in the behavior of the person. Our contention is that for training to succeed, instruction should adopt a model or process better equipped both to generate and to generalize appropriate responses.

The model proposed as an alternative is derived from the integrated-field psychology of J. R. Kantor, known as "interbehaviorism" (Kantor, 1976, 1980; Ruben, 1984b). This psychology defines the events of daily life as a constant interaction between human behavior, objects, and surrounding conditions through an indefinite number of life segments or *fields* (cf. Smith, 1973, 1984; Smith, Mountjoy, & Ruben, 1983). Interbehaviorism is fundamentally different from operant learning theory which says events and behavior can be reduced to instances of occurrence (cf. Morris, 1982, 1984). More than a theoretical distinction, this difference also explains why the training orientation accepts two basics about generalization. First, training is not a matter of simply teaching new skills to people. Rather, new skills are taught in the context of interactions with events. Second, skills learned under one situation do not "automatically" transfer to another situation. Instead, these skills progress through a series of successive situations (fields), all intricately connected and predictive of future assertive behavior.

An interbehavioral analysis of assertiveness training is discussed under two headings: "Teaching the person or behavior?" and "What does generalization mean?" Following this discussion is an outline of a model assertiveness workshop for managers incorporating both interbehavioral revisions.

Teaching the Person or Behavior?

Formal training in assertive communication skills has a long and profitable history beginning with the Dale Carnegie school in 1910. By 1930 the Carnegie school had expanded into a recognized educational institute promoting public speaking excellence. Pioneer efforts by A. Salter, J. Wolpe, and A. Lazarus further opened a vista of elaborate research opportunities, many of which currently expanded boundaries of assertiveness around a multidisciplinary framework. This increased with the commercial proliferation of assertiveness training in the form of groups or Assertiveness Skills Training Groups (ASTGs). ASTGs sprang up in droves and trainers developed highly complex behavioral profiles or physical descriptions of assertiveness. Descriptions consisted largely of verbal and nonverbal behaviors set in elaborate and creative definitions. Physical descriptions in their development and limitations lend contrast to a second definition called *functional descriptions*.

Physical Descriptions

Physical descriptions apparently strive for a content profile of assertiveness skills. Defined are all the major characteristics from "good" to "bad" forms of assertiveness behavior in the same way that one distinguishes a good dance step from a bad one. Clearly, written physical descriptions provide trainees with guidelines between hard and soft hand motions and, on a larger scale, between assertive and aggressive statements. Descriptions become more precise when they contain criteria to evaluate and monitor trainees. For example, criteria for relaxed gestures used by the authors in a recent workshop (Ruben, 1984a; Ruben & Ruben, 1985a) included:

1. Keep fingers spread apart about 2 mm.
2. Never point.
3. Start hand motions with palms and fingers turned toward the body and then "fan-out."
4. Never wrinkle forehead for longer than 30 sec.

Physical descriptions for these criteria delineate relaxed from tense hand gestures. Additional precision is brought about by assigning numerical values to each item for a single instance of the assertive response. For the third criterion, for instance, hand motions with palms and fingers turned toward the body and then fanned-out may have to occur for a certain number of times—say, twice. Details about the form of the response and how to measure it represent the defining features of most physical descriptions.

Given only physical descriptions, trainees in ASTGs will learn less about assertiveness than someone who learns to cook from reading a recipe. This is because recipes provide more than physical descriptions in the ingredients and additionally include interactions of these ingredients with appliances (events) around them. Training programs that include interactions serve to define not only what the behavior is but also how it operates on events in the environment. This operation or function of behavior becomes a critical variable when shifting the training perspective from the person to the behavior itself.

Functional Descriptions

Functional descriptions demystify the belief that assertive skills are internalized by intrapsychic dynamics and later manifest themselves in different situations. Leaders who exclude functional descriptions risk blaming training failures and errors on the trainees, trainers, or on the program design. Take an ASTG that produces trainees who apparently establish a better work attitude toward inter-personal employee relations. When these same graduates return to work, they find their positive attitudes diminish quickly and are replaced by previous forms of passivity. Typically they blame this relapse either on themselves, on leaders of the ASTG, or on certain feature of the training workshop. Self-imposed blame is particularly hazardous when the trainees are already passive or have doubts about their interpersonal skills. Women managers, for instance, may perceive this relapse as confirming their "inferiority to males" or start to believe ste-reotypes about women in business. Those managers more assured about their skills may instead blame their failures on inadequate instructors. Instructors are easy targets for criticism because they were responsible for the high risks and life-style changes to which trainees agreed under high expectations. When all else fails, criticism is directed at the instructional design. The structure or design of training lends itself to dissatisfaction depending on whether the ASTG was expensive, required enormous time commitments, or involved personal and emo-tional disclosures.

Another disadvantage from exclusive use of physical descriptions is the almost certain misconception of learning and performance. Are learning and perfor-mance the same thing, or do both represent distinct behavioral operations con-trolled by different environmental (stimulus) conditions? If they are distinct, then "learning" supposedly occurs when information is received or encoded as when hearing or reading instructions (i.e., following rules). When this information is decoded or expressed later under certain situations, the resultant behavior is said to be the "performance." Together, learning and performances would apparently account for assertive products. What the trainee gains from the ASTG would depend on his successful learning (not mastery) and subsequent display of the goals, objectives, and curricula during or after the program.

There is of course a problem with this distinction between learning and per-formance. On the one hand is the operant conditioning hypothesis (viz., radical behaviorism) arguing that learning and performance are the same, in that one must perform some contingent behaviors before knowledge (learning) of those contingencies can result. Skinner (1968) describes that "a student does not passively absorb knowledge from the world around him but must play an active role" (p. 5) to get knowledge and skills in curves of acquisition. Further reflection on this argument leads to a more confident conclusion: "Improved techniques have revealed an orderly relation between performance and contingencies and have eliminated the need to appeal to a separate inner learning process" (Skinner, 1974, p. 73).

Skinner's position regarding learning and performance would seem the solution to the artificial and problematic distinction found in most ASTG programming. However, in actual training the trials and errors of performance (acquisition) neither occur in isolated situations nor in an orderly fashion. Nor need learning be relegated the status of an "inner learning process." The "improved tech-niques" of which Skinner speaks are largely for the experimental analysis of behavior (in the laboratory), whereas when adapted for training use these techniques place unrealistic limits upon investigation. Such procedures "encourage the employment of mechanical and electrical analogies, making human beings into machines of various sorts, simple automata or complex computers" (Kantor, 1970, p. 103), rather than enabling an analysis of a larger inventory of factors.

These larger factors include the continuity of interrelated responses and stimulus objects. This "continuity" may be referred to as *learning interactions*. Over time, assertiveness responses are tried, produce consequences, encounter considerably different events, and all of this constitutes the learning process. Learning never occurs as a single transaction but is a function of multiple transactions. This means assertiveness skills taught in group today never are really learned today simply because the individual performed the skills correctly. All that can be predicted based on this sample of learning is the probability that performance may continue (or discontinue) given relatively unchanging circumstances. Predictions on future learning are called "interbehavioral potentials" (Ruben, 1983) and rely on functionally describing a more generous sample of conditions of behavior across settings.

To return to the criteria for relaxed hand gestures, a functional description amplified to cover more essential conditions of behavior might include these new items:

Behavior	Setting
1. Keep fingers spread apart about 2 mm.	When people are looking at you.
2. Never point.	When people are angry with you.
3. Start hand motions with palms . . .	When given a few minutes to talk.
4. Never wrinkle forehead . . .	In describing events that just happened or in showing surprise or dismay.

Notice under "setting" that nothing is mentioned about causes. Causality falsely implies that producing a behavior will automatically result in a single outcome. However, single causal outcomes are hard to identify because, in any given circumstance, there are many concurrent interactions (influences) upon behavior which have causal potential (Delprato, 1986; Ray & Brown, 1975; Sackett, 1979). Thus it becomes virtually impossible to single out one interaction as the primary cause. Alternatively, causal explanations are replaced by "potential setting events" that in the past have been present during successful assertive outcomes. The setting that corresponds to the first criterion, "When people are looking at you," describes the situation most predictable for reinforcing consequences. In short, adoption of functional descriptions in ASTGs better prepare the trainee for more realistic encounters beyond the training setting.

Figure 8.1
Diagram Depicting the Transfer of an Assertive Response from Training to Home-Related Settings, as Defined by the Concept of Stimulus Generalization.

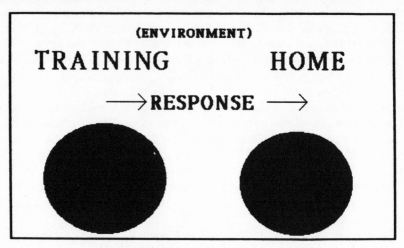

STIMULUS GENERALIZATION

What Does Generalization Mean?

While physical and functional descriptions refer primarily to the acquisitional phases, the next step is to teach assertiveness skills so they can transfer to events in the real world. Orthodox learning theory describes this transference of skills as a function of *generalization* (Pierrel, 1958). Skills are said to generalize when they reappear in the presence of same or similar events. This reappearance is known as *stimulus generalization* (cf. Kale, Kaye, Whelan, & Hopkins, 1968; Kirkland & Caughlin-Carver, 1982). "Stimulus generalization" is a prominent term in the assertive literature because the validity and reliability of ASTGs rely entirely on whether newly learned skills are reproduced in different settings, such as *from* training *to* the home setting (see Figure 8.1). Voice-control skills that appear only in the training setting, for example, lack generalization. Either the home setting lacks certain features or properties allowing assertiveness to transfer or the dimensions of assertiveness in training are different from this behavior at home.

What are these certain "dimensions of assertiveness"? Examined dimensions of assertive behavior may include response rate, frequency, duration, magnitude, latency, covariation, and setting events. For example, assertiveness training for victims of domestic violence may teach abilities in personal protection and in overcoming roadblocks. First the training begins in a contrived or simulated setting and then skills are tested in more realistic (in vivo) situations. Women who correctly follow the assertive model as taught in training are said to generalize this skill to their natural (home) environment.

The problem with this concept of generalization is that it assumes that the thing which transfers behavior is the person. Repeating the assertiveness under multiple settings may be a sign of generalization, but not if the ability to transfer this behavior supposedly lies within the person. Psychologists construct the concept of "repertoire" so they can talk about how behavior "stays within the person" when people interact in different situations (Ruben, 1983). The repertoire for this response is a misleading construct, adding to the misconception of the behavior functions. Rather than say the behavior "stays with the person," in interbehavioral trainers emphasize the interaction of this behavior with the environment. This is quite different from saying "people interact in different situations." That people interact in general is unimportant, but how they behave in those interactions determines whether new skills or old skills occur and produce reinforcing or punishing consequences.

In a way, behavior resides not within the person's repertoire but within the person's interaction with the environment—with the events around the person during his or her interaction. Since behavior and events are interactional, stimulus generalization assumes a new meaning. It means that behavior is not restricted to a specific situation but rather is continuous; it moves in and out of interactions along a continuum of fields, beginning at birth and ending at death. This continuum of fields contains the training setting and home (natural) setting. In each field of interaction the direction of cause is never unilateral, never a one-way influence as symbolically shown in traditional learning theory as S→ R. Interactions, instead, are bilateral or reciprocal and are represented by the two-headed arrow (↔) shown in figure 8.2. The sequence of interaction within each field and across fields provides for the inevitable progression of human learning over time. Field events also eliminate the need for regarding environmental setting as spatio-temporally distinct or mutually exclusive. This is simply an artificial distinction made when trainers think the training setting is different or separate from other settings appropriate for assertiveness.

The orthodox concept of stimulus generalization conflicts with the interbehavioral concept of field because of naturally occurring events. For instance, suppose a secretary learns in her assertiveness training class to "first ask about her supervisor's aggressive actions" before filing a grievance. Her assertiveness is demonstrated in every modeling and rehearsal exercise during the session. But that evening her husband returns home late from work and, in her perception, he is behaving aggressively. She immediately questions him for being late and an argument ensues; she gets "punished" for her initial assertive abilities. The following day at work this secretary endures her supervisor yelling at her. Without thinking, she goes to the personnel office and files a grievance against the supervisor. News of this grievance reaches the ASTG leader and the secretary returns to the program for "better generalization skills."

Ironically, had the incident at home not occurred, the secretary's skills might actually have generalized (in the Skinnerian sense). But this is an empirical question. Her training failed to encompass the most common or potential situ-

Figure 8.2
Diagram of Settings in a Continuous Sequence, Moving from Left to Right with the Passage of Time, Depicting the Event Interactions within and across Fields.

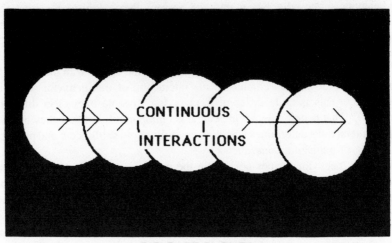

FIELD OF EVENTS
SEQUENCE OF INTERACTIONS

ations causing poor assertiveness. Instead, training concentrated only on the work-related setting and this never prepared the secretary for assertive behaviors at home. Functionally, the interactions at home were part of the larger field of events in that they followed in succession from the events of training. Without preparation for all the problematic situations in the trainee's life, skill generalization of any sort will fail regardless of the superb performance in training (cf. Ruben & Ruben, 1985b).

Interpretations of this field for assertiveness training must begin with two questions. First, what is the behavior in question? At this point, traditional learning theory and interbehavioral theory agree on defining verbal and nonverbal events as functional, not physical. Second, what are the potential interactions for this behavior or those that may cause a reinforcing outcome? Here the field theory is clearly unique with its reformulation of events as being continuous and not isolated. In planning an assertiveness course, both considerations would lay the foundation for realistic and lasting changes in assertive ability. The training model outlined below is a hypothetical example using those concepts in assertiveness programs for managers.

Training Model

Managers are offered a one-week comprehensive assertiveness training course. The newspaper advertisement states that managers can develop highly proficient assertiveness skills for work or home. The following sections give a brief overview of the course structure, goals, and objectives.

Goals and Objectives

Trainee goals are twofold. First, managers will learn to describe the behavior interactions. Second, managers will learn to use empathic "feeling words" according to the situation. Objectives consist of five parts. Managers will learn to describe (a) what preceded the event, (b) dimensions of behavior, (c) outcomes of the events, (d) functional interactions, and (e) basic feelings.

Structure

An initial evaluation of trainees is critical to later results. General assessment consists of direct behavioral observation on categories of verbal and nonverbal behaviors. Trainees watch videotaped scenes of potential assertive-employment situations and are asked to respond. Two recorders rate their replies based on degree of similarity or dissimilarity to a model reply, used in training the recorders. A single cue is used to alert trainees and recorders when to begin. Data from this assessment serve as part of the baseline record, supplemented by self-reports of poor assertiveness under two defined situations in the natural environment. One situation is whenever trainees feel insulted, offended, or angry. The second is whenever they feel tense, even though the antecedents to this emotion are inconspicuous or unknown. Reported situations from the natural environment later serve as the basis for simulated or in vivo rehearsals, also videotaped and reviewed. Then trainees will watch playbacks of the videotape and learn about potential interactions for functionally describing what preceded the event, behavior, and its outcomes.

One week later, intervention begins. Techniques such as modeling, token economy, behavioral rehearsal, homework assignments, and audiovideo feedback are used during lessons. Lessons follow components of verbal and nonverbal behavior using confederates or significant others selected from the natural environment or from wherever assertive deficits (excesses) reportedly occur. The token economy system in abbreviated form simply includes a point availability for correct homework assignment (completion) and accurate imitations during test trials. Later points are awarded for trials in all targeted *and nontargeted* settings in the natural environment. Points accumulated per session are redeemed either for adult gifts (magazines, grocery coupons, sports tickets) or for work privileges (comp time, longer lunch, and so on).

Outcome Assessment

Following scheduled training, plans are needed to determine continuity of the learned skills into the natural environment. Posttherapy assessment is actually "put into action" long before the training ends. Initially, trainees agree to participate in follow-up observations scheduled on four different dates: three, six, nine, and twelve months away. Part of the training fee (e.g., $10) is refunded for attendance on each of the follow-up dates. For example, ten dollars is rebated on each of the four dates if the trainee shows up and submits to observational assessment.

The observational test resembles that used during baseline (videotape) but also includes a test where the trainee describes and demonstrates skills in nontargeted situations from the natural environment. Recorded on videotape are the accuracy and similarity of the trainee's replies. Where skill deficits or excesses are still indicated, that refunded money ($10) can be used toward another, individually scheduled training session.

Analysis of Training Model

This brief example describes only one, among many, conceivable procedures to assure that assertiveness skills in the acquisition, maintenance, and follow-up phases conform to a field approach. Clinical interventions for group assertiveness that include videotape recordings or simulations ("analogues") additionally cover interactions that otherwise are inaccessible to the trainer in the classroom. Events at work or home are further represented by self-reports or by audiotaped records. Toward this same goal, homework assignments directly stress applications of new behavior in *interaction with different potential events* that already exist in the trainees' lives.

Summary

Today's heralded success of assertiveness-training programs ignores critical assumptions in the training techniques. Failures in assertiveness outside the training environment remain unrecognized because trainers nearly always observe successful performance *during* the training session. This neglect of comprehensive training is due to two basic assumptions in program philosophy. First, the training orientation assumes that information passes from the training setting into "real" settings because of some intrapsychic dynamic within the trainee. Learning theorists inadvertently enhance this assumption by saying that behavior resides in a person's repertoire, although this repertoire is by no means "inside" the person. Second, training orientations assume that behavior learned in one setting will automatically transfer to new settings provided that the procedures in these settings are replicated.

In contrast to these assumptions is the interbehavioral or integrated-field approach that emphasizes two alternative ways to ensure efficacy of assertiveness programs. First, assertive behaviors make sense when they are described as interactions with events around them. The description is a functional description. And second, training must extend beyond the group session given that a person's interactions do not occur in isolated situations, but rather through a continuous flow of successive events.

References

Alberti, R. E. (Ed.) 1977. *Assertiveness: Innovations, applications, issues*. San Luis Obispo, Calif.: Impact Publishers.

Brown, S. D., and L. W. Brown. 1980. Trends in assertion training research and practice: A content analysis of the published literature. *Journal of Clinical Psychology*, 36: 265–69.

Delprato, D. J. 1986. Response patterns. In H. W. Reese and L. J. Parrott (eds.), *Advances in behavioral science*. Hillside, N.J.: Lawrence Erlbaum Associates.

Galassi, M. D., and J. P. Galassi. 1978. Assertion: a critical review. *Psychotherapy* 15: 16–29.

Kale, R. J., J. H. Kaye, P. A. Whelan, and B. L. Hopkins. 1968. The effects of reinforcement on the modification, maintenance, and generalization of social responses of mental patients. *Journal of Applied Behavior Analysis* 1: 307–14.

Kantor, J. R. 1970. An analysis of the experimental analysis of behavior (TEAB). *Journal of the Experimental Analysis of Behavior* 15: 101–8.

Kantor, J. R. 1976. The origin and evolution of interbehavioral psychology. *Revista Mexicano de Analsis de la Conducta* 2: 120–36.

Kantor, J. R. 1980. Manifesto of interbehavioral psychology. *Revista Mexicano de Analisis de la Conducta* 6: 117–28.

Kirkland, K., and J. Caughlin-Carver. 1982. Maintenance and generalization of assertive skills. *Education and Training of the Mentally Retarded* 17: 313–18.

Lange, A. J., D. C. Rimm, and J. Loxley. 1975. Cognitive-behavioral assertion training procedures. *Counseling Psychologist* 5: 37–41.

Morris, E. K. 1982. Some relationships between interbehavioral psychology and radical behaviorism. *Behaviorism* 10: 187–216.

Morris, E. K. 1984. Interbehavioral psychology and radical behaviorism: Some similarities and differences. *The Behavior Analyst* 7: 197–204.

Pierrel, R. 1958. A generalization gradient for auditory intensity in the rat. *Journal of the Experimental Analysis of Behavior* 1: 303–13.

Rathus, S. A. 1975. Principles and practices of assertion training: An eclectic overview. *Counseling Psychology* 5: 9–20.

Ray, R., and D. Brown. 1975. A systems approach to behavior. *Psychological Record* 25: 459–78.

Ruben, D. H. 1983. Interbehavioral implications for behavior therapy: Clinical perspectives. In N. W. Smith, P. T. Mountjoy, and D. H. Ruben (Eds.), *Reassessment in psychology: The interbehavioral alternative*. Washington, D.C.: University Press of America.

Ruben, D. H. 1984a. Comparison of two analogue measures for assessing and teaching assertiveness to physically disabled elderly: An exploratory study. *Gerontology and Geriatric Education* 5: 63–71.

Ruben, D. H. 1984b. Major trends in interbehavioral psychology from articles published in the *Psychological Record* (1973–1983). *Psychological Record* 34: 589–617.

Ruben D. H. 1985. *Progress in assertiveness, 1973–1983: An analytical bibliography.* Metuchen, N.J.: Scarecrow Press.

Ruben, D. H. and M. J. Ruben. 1985a. Interviewing skills: Implications for vocation counseling with alcoholic clients. *Alcoholism Treatment Quarterly* 1: 133–40.

Ruben, D. H. and M. J. Ruben. 1985b. *Sixty seconds to success.* Bradenton, Fl.: Pine Mountain Press.

Sackett, G. P. 1979. The lag sequential analysis of contingency and cyclicity in behavioral interaction research. In J. D. Osofsky (Ed.), *Handbook of infant development.* New York: Wiley.

Skinner, B. F. 1968. *The technology of teaching.* New York: Appleton-Century-Crofts.

Skinner, B. F. 1974. *About behaviorism.* New York: Vintage.

Smith, N. W. 1973. Interbehavioral psychology: Roots and branches. *Psychological Record* 23: 157–67.

Smith, N. W. 1984. Fundamentals of interbehavioral psychology. *Psychological Record* 34: 479–94.

Smith, N.W., P. T. Mountjoy, and D. H. Ruben. 1983. *Reassessment in psychology: The interbehavioral alternative.* Washington, D.C.: University Press of America.

Whiteley, J. and J. V. Flowers. 1978. *Approaches to assertion training.* Belmont, Calif.: Brooks/Cole.

9

Multidisciplinary Approach to Obesity and Risk-Factor Management

Dallas W. Stevenson and Michael J. Hemingway

More than ten years ago, A. J. Stunkard (1975) characterized traditional treatment of obesity as grossly ineffectual. He contrasted it with a radically different and apparently very effective "behavioral approach." More recently, however, A. J. Stunkard and S. B. Pennick (1979) have questioned the clinical significance of the behavioral approach to the treatment of obesity. Failure of behavior therapy to achieve and maintain clinically significant reductions in weight have led to criticisms of orthodox behavioral practices. The observation that groups treated for obesity either fail to lose weight or regain weight following treatment (Brownell, 1982) has prompted an increase in vitalistic and animistic explanations from researchers in the field. An interbehavioral perspective offers an alternative to regressions of scientific thinking in obesity research and treatment. This chapter will contrast the interbehavioral perspective to other approaches with specific references to set-point theory. Further, we will describe two service delivery systems influenced by the interbehavioral perspective.

From Set Point to Field-Factor Analysis

One of the most prominent approaches to obesity research and treatment today is referred to as "set-point theory." This section will introduce the reader to applications of the set-point notion to obesity; it is a brief discussion of set-point theory (although a detailed analysis would clearly benefit the field).

Researchers have used the term set point in several ways (Mrosovsky & Powley, 1977). These uses include (a) as an explanatory construct in the framework of linear mechanics or the statistical-correlational stage of scientific thinking (Kantor, 1946) and (b) as a constructive description consistent with the integrated-field or systems approach to science (Kantor, 1953). K. D. Brownell's (1982) account exemplifies set-point theory in the former sense, according to which each individual's body has a set point for weight and the body will struggle to protect any deviation from this personal ideal weight. Proponents of this view often indicate that the set point is somehow inscribed in the individual's central nervous system or some other physiological structure. A hypothetical "pounderstat" or perhaps a "lipidstat" or "glucostat" forces the organism to engage in activity that defends this ideal weight. According to Brownell (1982), "some obese persons may be fighting a battle with biology that never relents" (p. 822). He then goes on to quote W. Bennet and J. Gurin's (1982) view of the obese person's attempt to overcome the set point: "It is not a fair contest. The set point is a tireless opponent. The dieter's only allies are willpower and whatever incentives there are that make chronic physical discomfort worthwhile" (p. 822). Brownell's (1982) and Bennet and Gurin's (1982) position resurrects the traditions of reductionism, dualism, and vitalism. It inhibits systematic study by ascribing causes to unobservable entities within the organism.

What might the course of action be for the researcher or clinician? Choices might include (a) undertaking crash program to locate the pounderstat so that drugs and surgery might be used to alter the faulty mechanism, (b) enhancing willpower and incentives so the obese individuals can endure "chronic physical discomfort," or (c) indicating that obese persons must learn to live with their condition and that the research clinician is going into smoking cessation.

J.E.R. Staddon (1983) uses the set-point notion as a constructive descriptor to explain the interaction of various observed events on eating behavior from a systems perspective. According to Staddon's version, in any system there are various subsystems that have optimal ranges of functioning which vary with participating subsystem changes and these systems are constantly adapting toward optimal functioning ranges.

Staddon's view is compatible with contemporary integrated-field theory, and it prompts the scientist to investigate and describe the relationship between events over time. This stands in sharp contrast to the reductionistic version of set-point theory in which culturally transmitted constructs are impressed on the data. The systems or field-factor approach has broad implications for treatment and intervention in obesity.

P. R. Fuller (1983) nicely states a major consideration that calls for systems analysis: "When one moves from the most simple type of relationships one discovers that almost everything is multidetermined, . . . there are many factors which interact in many different ways in order to attain a particular result" (p. 1). Figure 9.1 attempts to represent some of the major interacting factors that are of particular relevance in the area of obesity and health. Health is depicted as a complex state of the organism in constant interaction with a wide range of interrelated systemic factors evolving across time. The field-factor approach helps the scientist-practitioner confront the multitude of biological and psychological factors one encounters in obesity and risk-factor management. The systemic view

Figure 9.1
Field Factors Related to Health

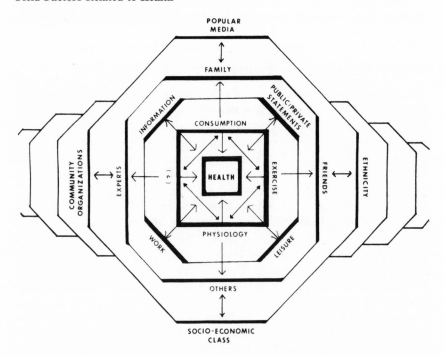

of obesity leads us to take data on body composition, blood pressure, lipids, and other measures of organismic functioning, rather than focusing on weight alone. We examine consumption patterns and composition of intake rather than a single measure such as Kcal/day. Instead of citing insufficient willpower we examine cultural, familial, and personal interaction patterns.

The work of P. C. Mackeen, B. A. Franklin, W. C. Nicholas, and E. R. Buskirk (1983) serves as one rather simple but elegant example of (a) problems encountered when a single factor (for example, weight) is used to evaluate treatment outcomes and (b) the interaction of factors in the treatment of obesity. Loss of body fat rather than lean tissue, water, or other constituents is viewed as one very important target outcome in obesity programs. Mackeen and colleagues were interested in investigating the outcome obtained during caloric restriction when exercise parameters were varied and percent body fat and weight were recorded. The percentage of weight loss due to decreases in body fat covaried with changes in the level of exercise such that without aerobic exercise only 10 percent of weight loss was body fat, whereas at moderate levels of aerobic exercise as much as 80 percent of the weight lost was body fat.

Intervention in obesity, therefore, involves the description of the participating factors, their interrelationships across time, and the identification of trajectories which are indicative of health and of disease. Furthermore, intervention requires determination of which factors need to be altered and what techniques are most effective at altering these factors in order to deflect problematic trajectories (Delprato & McGlynn, 1986).

Guidelines for Obesity Treatment Programs

A field-factor analysis leads to a rather complex picture, even in the simplified cases. To develop a treatment approach from this perspective requires the delineation of constructional guidelines. Starting from an interbehavioral perspective, D. J. Delprato and F. D. McGlynn (1986) have formulated a set of six postulates for behavioral medicine. Using these postulates and pertinent research findings, we offer the following guidelines for obesity treatment programs.

1. *FIELD POSTULATE: The Events of Behavioral Medicine Are Comprised of Multifactor Fields.* The focus of treatment and research in obesity is the interaction of individuals with objects and events. This suggests that instrumentation and patient record systems must be developed to describe an event-field composed of contextual setting conditions, media of stimulation (light, air), and the organic state of the individual. Thus, constructs must be based on systematic observations of these interactions, not explanations derived from dualistic or mentalistic traditions.

2. *HOLISTIC POSTULATE: The Entire Organism, Not Only Specific Components, Participates in Its Performance.* This postulate suggests that clinicians recognize that the activities of obese patients involve the whole organism. Thus, dualism and physiological and biological reductionism are rejected. Rather than being viewed as the basis for obesity, biological structures and functions are viewed as *participating field factors*.

3. *EVOLUTIONAL POSTULATE: Behavioral Medicine Works with Multifactor Fields That Have Evolved or Are Evolving.* Vitalistic and mechanistic explanations so prevalent in obesity literature are unnecessary when the behavior of the obese patient is viewed as the outcome of ongoing biosocial evolution. The obese client's functioning is a naturalistic outcome of a continuous stream of developmental processes.

4. *INTERDISCIPLINARY POSTULATE: The Practice of Behavioral Medicine Demands Interdisciplinary Cooperation.* Many fields have developed specialized techniques for addressing participating field factors in obesity. In order to intervene effectively, a transdisciplinary team composed of experts from many fields must work in concert to determine and achieve treatment objectives. No discipline is viewed as more basic than any other. On some occasions one discipline may receive more emphasis than others, depending on the relative contribution of specific field factors.

5. *TACTICAL POSTULATE: Clinical Procedures Are Seen as Modifications of Field Factors.* Therapy, management, research, and prevention in obesity consist of systematic study and modification of factors in a multifactor field

including, as needed, the biological, social, domestic, economic, educational, and vocational factors participating in the patient's life.

6. *GOAL POSTULATE: The Goals of Behavioral Medicine Are Alterations in Developmental Trajectories.* Continuous development is a central concept of a field perspective. Examination of the individual's developmental history is useful in projecting future development, or describing developmental trajectories. The goal of treatment is to manipulate critical field factors; this creates a deflection of established trajectories. Thus the goal of research and treatment in obesity and risk-factor management is to identify and manipulate critical field factors in order to deflect developmental trajectories away from disease/dysfunction to health and well-being.

These postulates upon which we base our guidelines have several clear implications for development of service delivery systems for obesity and risk-factor management. First, the field-factor and evolutional postulates require that practitioners develop data systems capable of tracking several variables for an individual over time. In order to ascertain the relative participation of various field factors, new analytical techniques (perhaps time-series analysis similar to that described by Gottman, 1981) will have to replace current reliance on time-independent statistics. The multidisciplinary postulate requires that nutritionists, physicians, physiologists, psychologists, pathologists, and members of other disciplines work in concert to select variables to be measured and appropriate measurement techniques for the assessment of clinical strategy. The goal postulates suggest that intervention and measurement must be long-term (clearly a deflection of body fat, blood glucose, or problematic eating for two weeks fails to meet the goal of maintaining a health trajectory). The tactical postulate suggests that obesity and risk-factor management intervene in several systems using several techniques. Thus, the service delivery system may include didactic lecture, training, exercises, contingency management, and feedback of process and product goals. The program should involve not only the identified participant but also family members, friends, coworkers, educational systems, and other systems the identified client contacts directly or indirectly. Finally, the postulates suggest that the service providers in the service delivery system should adapt their activities to systematic interactions with product and process data. Thus, the service delivery system should be in a continuous state of guided evolution toward more efficacious intervention rather than constant adaptation to noncritical aspects of the cultural context.

The Obesity and Risk Factor Program at Wayne State University

The Obesity and Risk Factor Program (ORFP) at Wayne State University has experienced some success by employing many of the previously mentioned notions in its mission to conduct treatment and research for obesity and risk factors (Taylor, Stevenson, Dulmage, & Lucas, 1985). In 1975, A. J. Stunkard noted that most who entered treatment for obesity did not stay in treatment, most who stayed did not lose weight, and those who lost weight did not keep it off. N. K. Holmes, E. A. Ardito, D. W. Stevenson, and C. P. Lucas (1984) reported that most individuals who entered the ORFP at Wayne State University stayed in treatment. The authors further reported that patients treated at the clinic lost an average of 58 pounds, with a range of from 14 to 212 pounds, and that approximately 56.8 percent maintained the loss at one-year follow-up.

The ORFP utilizes a long-term, multimodal approach to the treatment of obesity. The staff includes professionals in medicine, behavioral science, nutrition, exercise, physiology, nursing, statistical analysis, computer programming, and administration. Further, the clinic employs several support staff including data technicians, bookkeepers, medical technicians, secretaries, and research assistants. Clients are individuals who are at least 40 pounds over ideal weight and exhibit risk factors (elevated blood pressure, glucose, cholesterol, and so on). The current program is outlined in Figure 9.2. It uses system interventions, including several derived from behavior therapy, and a medically monitored protein-sparing modified fast. As indicated in the figure, the client completes a sequential program whose major phases consist of prefasting, fasting, refeeding, and maintenance.

Our systems orientation leads us to use a variety of methods to contact potential program participants. The ORFP professional staff participates in a community education program that consists of lectures to community organizations, radio and television appearances, and presentations at professional meetings. ORFP professionals also are encouraged to contribute to the clinic newsletter, local newspapers, and professional journals. Current and former clients of the program frequently prompt family and friends to approach the ORFP. Finally, marketing representatives contact area physicians in an effort to establish referral sources.

Phase A: Prefasting

The prefasting segment spans approximately eight weeks; it provides the opportunity for assessment and prepares the individual for subsequent phases of the program.

The orientation is the initial meeting in Phase A. The professional staff, including a clinic physician, psychologists, and nurse-administrator, introduce and describe the program. A brief history of the treatment of obesity, the development of the protein-sparing modified fast, and clinical results are outlined. The notion of assessing one's "life-style" and the subsequent long-term modification of it are discussed. The specific phases of the program are described as are the responsibilities of the client. The client is instructed to begin collecting data on food intake and exercise. A checkbook-type record-keeping system is utilized. The time, location, food consumed, and exercise performed is noted in the record book. Required attendance and future homework assignments are stressed. At the conclusion of orientation, clients interested in participating in

Figure 9.2

Obesity and Risk Factor Program at Wayne State University

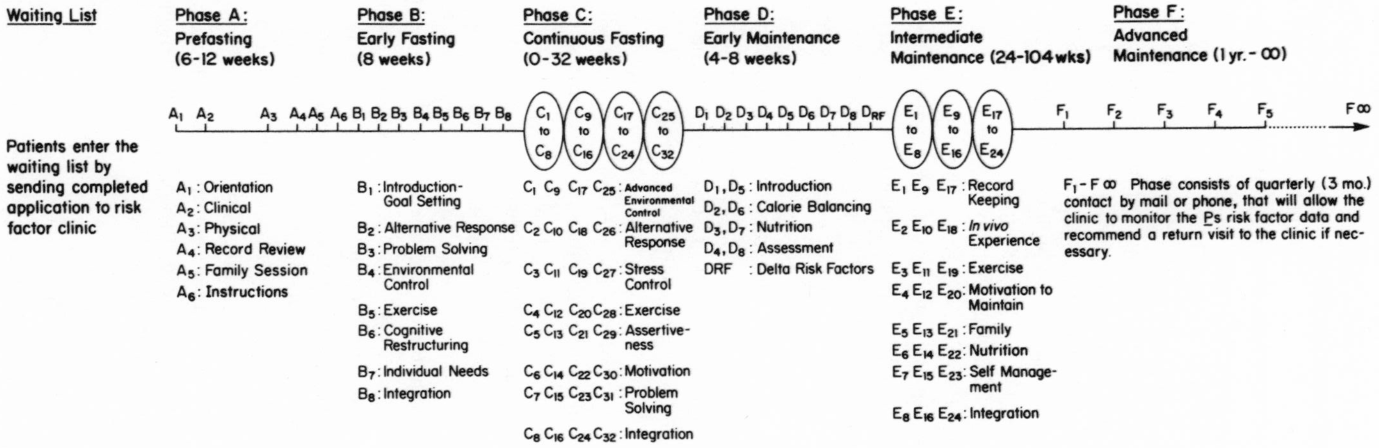

Waiting List	Phase A: Prefasting (6-12 weeks)	Phase B: Early Fasting (8 weeks)	Phase C: Continuous Fasting (0-32 weeks)	Phase D: Early Maintenance (4-8 weeks)	Phase E: Intermediate Maintenance (24-104 wks)	Phase F: Advanced Maintenance (1 yr.- ∞)

Timeline: A_1 A_2 A_3 $A_4 A_5$ A_6 B_1 B_2 B_3 B_4 B_5 B_6 B_7 B_8 (C_1 to C_8) (C_9 to C_{16}) (C_{17} to C_{24}) (C_{25} to C_{32}) D_1 D_2 D_3 D_4 D_5 D_6 D_7 D_8 D_{RF} (E_1 to E_8) (E_9 to E_{16}) (E_{17} to E_{24}) F_1 F_2 F_3 F_4 F_5 F_∞

Patients enter the waiting list by sending completed application to risk factor clinic

Phase A:
A_1 : Orientation
A_2 : Clinical
A_3 : Physical
A_4 : Record Review
A_5 : Family Session
A_6 : Instructions

Phase B:
B_1 : Introduction-Goal Setting
B_2 : Alternative Response
B_3 : Problem Solving
B_4 : Environmental Control
B_5 : Exercise
B_6 : Cognitive Restructuring
B_7 : Individual Needs
B_8 : Integration

Phase C:
C_1, C_9, C_{17}, C_{25} : Advanced Environmental Control
$C_2, C_{10}, C_{18}, C_{26}$: Alternative Response
$C_3, C_{11}, C_{19}, C_{27}$: Stress Control
$C_4, C_{12}, C_{20}, C_{28}$: Exercise
$C_5, C_{13}, C_{21}, C_{29}$: Assertiveness
$C_6, C_{14}, C_{22}, C_{30}$: Motivation
$C_7, C_{15}, C_{23}, C_{31}$: Problem Solving
$C_8, C_{16}, C_{24}, C_{32}$: Integration

Phase D:
D_1, D_5 : Introduction
D_2, D_6 : Calorie Balancing
D_3, D_7 : Nutrition
D_4, D_8 : Assessment
DRF : Delta Risk Factors

Phase E:
E_1, E_9, E_{17} : Record Keeping
E_2, E_{10}, E_{18} : In vivo Experience
E_3, E_{11}, E_{19} : Exercise
E_4, E_{12}, E_{20} : Motivation to Maintain
E_5, E_{13}, E_{21} : Family
E_6, E_{14}, E_{22} : Nutrition
E_7, E_{15}, E_{23} : Self Management
E_8, E_{16}, E_{24} : Integration

Phase F:
$F_1 - F_\infty$ Phase consists of quarterly (3 mo.) contact by mail or phone, that will allow the clinic to monitor the P's risk factor data and recommend a return visit to the clinic if necessary.

the program meet with support personnel to make an appointment for the next meeting.

Clinical and physical examinations follow. Submaximal exercise stress tests and hydrostatic weighing are completed by exercise physiologists. The medical component of the treatment program provides the initial and ongoing analysis of detected risk factors. Following the physical, clients are given an appointment for the family session.

The "family session" provides the opportunity for clinic members and their friends and family to discuss potentially problematic situations for fasting persons and the people around them. Two staff psychologists direct the group. During the first exercise, the clinic members and their guests work in small groups discussing situations that may be problematic during the fast. Possible solutions are then presented, and the psychologists offer feedback in an attempt to shape responses. The individuals are then given a "Family Trouble-Shooting Manual" developed by the staff psychologists. The manual provides recommended solutions to typical problems fasting individuals encounter. Examples of pertinent issues are environmental control, establishing reciprocal relationships as opposed to the client functioning in the sick role, and finding alternatives to consumption. Clients and their support group are asked to incorporate this process into their home life.

The "record review" was designed as an opportunity for the psychologists to further instruct incoming clients in the record-keeping procedure required once beginning the fast. Further, there is discussion of the client's observations of patterns in consumption and exercise. An "eating inventory," a checklist reflective of these patterns, is completed. An exercise in the form of seven days of blank records, entitled "imaginary fast," prompts clients to examine when and where they will exercise and take the prescribed supplement to the fast and allows the practice of the energy balance computation procedure. The clients are also presented with a list of prefasting assignments. They are instructed to continue collecting data on food intake and exercise and to begin walking on a minimal basis with their physician's permission. They are to continue to note patterns in consumption and experiment with alternative patterns. And finally, they are to plan alternative activities to consumption to commence with the fast.

The final prefasting meeting involves various instructions. The physician, psychologist, and nurse-administrator once again address the group. The physician details each client's diagnosis and answers any questions. The nurse-administrator provides verbal and written instructions regarding the taking of the supplement. The psychologist utilizes this time to review client follow-through on assignments, answer questions, and make recommendations. ORFP members are given a brief test of the basic instructions presented by the nurse-administrator. The fast typically begins the next day.

Phase B: Early Fasting

Phase B is an eight-week segment. Clients meet with a physician weekly, have their blood pressure and weight measured weekly, and have their blood drawn biweekly. Clients are required to meet with the physician in order to purchase the protein supplement. Psychologists also meet clients weekly in a group session which lasts an hour and a half. The data collection system requires the client to turn in to the psychologist the prior week's records of food intake and caloric expenditure. A summary sheet is also completed by the client. At the next meeting the psychologist returns it to the client with written feedback. The psychologist asks all clients to report the number of days they kept records and exercised and the total exercise calories for the week. The prior week's topic and homework assignment are briefly reviewed, and the week's topic is presented. Topics discussed include goal setting, alternative response training, problem solving, environmental control, exercise, and cognitive restructuring. At week eight the client completes a written test of the Phase B topics. The clients also complete an evaluation of the phase.

Phase C: Continued Fasting

Those individuals who do not achieve their goal weight at the end of Phase B enter Phase C (continue fasting). The client maintains the same schedule of interaction with the clinic. Additional topics are presented, with prior ones addressed in greater detail. During the fasting stage of the program, the emphasized goal is complete fasting. The ongoing instruction in the analysis of significant field factors and in the application of specific intervention strategies contribute to the attainment of this goal.

Phase D: Early Maintenance

When individuals have successfully attained their stated goals, or at the recommendation of the ORFP team, the client enters early maintenance. This phase is eight weeks in length. The group format is used as before, except that a dietician directs the group. Clients continue to have consultative access to psychologists. The initial focus is on preparing the fasting person for the refeeding process (they continue to fast completely during weeks one and two). The introduction of food is accomplished systematically and results in an increase in caloric intake to the maintenance level. The refeeding process involves fading the supplements and replacing them with prescribed meals. Physician contact is discontinued after the fourth week due to a consumption schedule of 800 calories per day and two prescribed meals plus supplement. Blood pressure and weight continue to be measured weekly. Blood is drawn biweekly through week four, during the eighth or last week of early maintenance, and every three months thereafter. During the group session, specific topics are presented and objectives outlined. Clients are taught several methods of analyzing their eating, including: (a) composition, or determination of the relative proportions of major nutrients as well as the vitamin and mineral content in the food they are eating; (b) caloric volume, the amount of calories in food; (c) caloric rate, the rate at which they consume calories during a specific eating episode; and (d) pattern of eating, or the number of hours between eating. Program participants are taught the relationship between their eating patterns and their treatment objectives. At the conclusion of Phase D, clients are required to develop a personal eating plan.

Risk—Factor Review

Directly after the last Phase D meeting and preceding the first Phase E meeting all clients attend a risk-factor review with the clinic medical director. During this meeting client progress is reviewed and the clinic medical director restates the importance of maintaining new patterns of consumption and activity necessary to support treatment gains.

Phase E: Intermediate Maintenance

Following the risk-factor review the client moves into a maintenance group, or Phase E. The group is directed by a psychologist; however, the client still has the opportunity to consult with a dietician. Clients are requested to attend clinic weekly for a miminum of six months, with no maximum time limit. Throughout this phase participants continue to be responsible for their own menu planning. Group topics include many of those presented during prior phases, with the emphasis upon how these topics and skills are pertinent to an individual striving to maintain treatment results. Based on the report authored by Holmes and colleagues (1984), the clinic emphasizes record keeping, calorie counting, exercise, and clinic attendance during this period. The goal of an individual during the maintenance stage is to maintain his or her goal weight, blood pressure, blood lipid levels, blood sugar level, size and other products of his or her participation in the clinic program. In the maintenance period, the client takes the role of analyst and assumes primary responsibility for ongoing analyses of the significant field factors. It becomes the client's responsibility to observe, to record eating and movement, to note how these activities approximate performance standards necessary to maintain the benefits derived from fasting, and to make adjustments in these activities or factors that affect these activities when necessary.

Phase F: Advanced Maintenance

When clients have mastered maintenance performance skills or they decide to discontinue weekly group participation, they move to advanced maintenance. There is quarterly contact with the individual by telephone or mail, thus continuing the monitoring process.

Client Data System

A major goal of the treatment system is to facilitate the development of a data information system that yields continuous feedback on client progress. The current methodology employs an eating and activity log that resembles a checkbook. Clients are taught to record the date, time, location, type, and amount of food or activity and the effect of the food intake or activity on their energy balance. To teach clients the impact of eating and exercising they are instructed to deposit the amount of calories they have to spend (the amount calculated to maintain current weight) in their log. When they take in calories they are taught to subtract from this balance; when they exercise they add calories to the balance. A negative balance indicates that the client is in positive energy balance and storing fat; a zero balance signals equal energy balance and maintenance of current fat stores. A positive balance shows the client is in negative energy balance and is burning stored fat. Because 3,500 calories are stored in a pound of fat, clients can always predict the impact of their current eating and exercise on fat storage. For example, a balance of $-3,500$, 0, and $+3,500$ predicts a gain of one pound of fat, no change in fat, and a loss of one pound, respectively. To provide calibration of this system, clients are taught to measure and record variables indicative of treatment progress. They are taught to record predicted weight (based on log data), actual scale weight, and girth measurement on a weekly basis. Each month clients adjust their calculations so that their log accurately predicts changes in the other treatment measures. Finally, the client's personal data system contains several variables that the client and psychologist agree represent objective measures of treatment goals. Once the client data system is contructed, the client takes responsibility for maintenance of the system (including making and recording scheduled measurements).

The ORFP attempts to promote maintenance of the client data system by collecting the products of the system, offering clients opportunities to discuss the products of the system, and by publishing (in ORFP newsletter and professional publications) data describing the relationship between maintaining the personal data system and clinic measures of treatment.

ORFP Data System

The client data system was designed to function as a compass, giving the clients critical feedback on their position with respect to their goals. The computerized ORFP data system, represented in Figure 9.3, integrates several key systemic factors, including clients, their families, referring physicians, ORFP staff, ORFP laboratories, exercise laboratory, and the client data system. The system is designed to give feedback on critical treatment variables to many participants in the ORFP systems, to provide systematic consequences to the clinic personnel for changes in treatment variables, and to provide a data base capable of generating answers to basic and applied research questions.

Several treatment variables including weight, systolic blood pressure, total cholesterol, HDL cholesterol, blood sugar, triglycerides, pulse rate, basal metabolic rate, body composition, functional aerobic impairment, ORFP attendance, calories consumed, exercise, and days of completed eating and activity log are

Figure 9.3
Clinic Data System

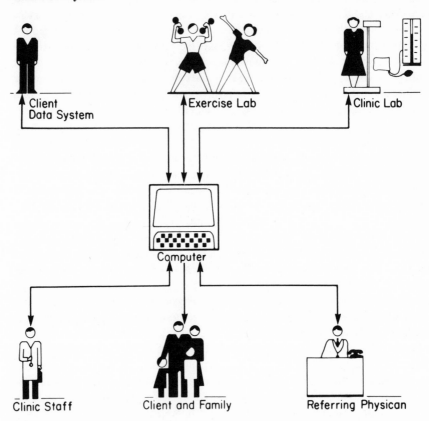

entered into the ORFP data base. At regular intervals the ORFP computer produces reports detailing changes in these variables for each of the clients in the
program. Irrespective of the direction of the change, reports are delivered to the
client, the client's referring physician, and the clinic staff. Data collection begins
with the first clinic contact and continues through all phases of the program.
Thus, not only does the system provide systematic feedback to participants in
the clinic (both clients and the service providers), it also provides feedback to
the ORFP's referral base. This consequence makes it important for the ORFP
survival that treatment becomes effective in altering these variables in the desired
direction.

In the field of obesity and risk-factor management there are many controversies
regarding both treatment objectives and methodology for obtaining those objectives. At the same time there is a notable paucity of systematic long-term data
regarding these questions. The data system was designed to guide the evolution

of clinic objectives and methods. Its purpose is to ensure that the inevitable changes in the program are adaptations to systematic observations of treatment objectives and not vague notions regarding objectives or methodology.

Summary of Outcome Data of the ORFP

This section summarizes some outcome data yielded by the ORFP data system. Holmes and colleagues (1984) examined weight loss and weight maintenance for 127 participants in the ORFP. Participants lost between 14 and 212 pounds, with an average loss of 58 pounds. Further, 56.8 percent of participants maintained their weight loss at one year follow-up and participants who maintained their personal data system and continued to exercise regained significantly less weight than those who did not.

N. Ahmad, H. Yee, D. Stevenson, S. Taylor, N. Holmes, L. Darga, T. Spafford, and C. Lucas (1985) examined blood pressure changes in ORFP participants who completed Phases A through D and at least six months of Phase E. Blood pressure showed significant reductions from the first Phase A visit to the last visit of Phase D, with mean systolic blood pressure dropping 14.4 mmHg (range 10 to 24 mmHg) and mean diastolic blood pressure dropping 11 mmHg (range 10 to 18 mmHg). At six months into Phase E, blood pressure remained significantly lower than Phase A measurements, with mean systolic blood pressure remaining 7 mmHg (range 9.3 to 17.5 mmHg) lower and mean diastolic remaining 8 mmHg (range 17 to 20 mmHg) lower. Ahmad and colleagues also found that hypertensive participants achieved and maintained significantly greater blood pressure reductions than normotensive participants.

Lucas, Stevenson, Darga, Yee, Ahmad, Holmes, Taylor, S. Kasim, and Spafford (1985) studied serum lipid changes in participants who completed Phases A through D and at least six months of Phase E. They reported maintenance of significant reductions of LDL-cholesterol (LDL-C), with mean LDL-C remaining 16.1 mg/dl lower than Phase A levels. Lucas et al. also noted achievement and maintenance of a significant increase in HDL-cholesterol (HDL-C) with mean HDL-C remaining 10.6 mg/dl higher than Phase A levels. This contributed to a significant decrease in total cholesterol (TC) to HDL-C ratio, with the mean TC/HDL-C ratio remaining 1.2 mg/dl lower than Phase A measurement and indicating decreased risk of cardiovascular disease.

Finally, in a study demonstrating notable improvements in body composition and fitness, B. A. Franklin and J. Scherf (1985) examined changes in those variables from Phase A to Phase E in six participants. Hydrostatic weighing revealed a decrease in mean percentage of body fat, from 37.64 (range 47.4 to 29.5) to 24.78 (range 30.3 to 14.1). Maximal exercise testing demonstrated a decrease in functional aerobic impairment, from a mean percentage of impairment of 34.8 (range 52 to 17) to 13 (range 43 to -23).

The Healthy Life Program

The Healthy Life Program (HLP) emerged from the question of how to establish a service delivery network that would address (a) severe cases of obesity, (b) less severe cases of obesity, (c) cases which involve low but developing risks (not necessarily obesity), and (d) maintenance of altered ("healthier") life-styles. The ORFP was attending to (d) and did have a carefully developed maintenance program, but there remained a need for a program based closer to the community of ORFP participants, one which deemphasized weight loss and focused on healthy eating and exercise as the critical goals. Professional staff from the ORFP and the Birmingham (Michigan) YMCA were organized to develop such a program.

The HLP was offered at the YMCA as a specialized service to members only. It was sponsored by the ORFP, thus creating a community-based program sponsored by reputable and well-known organizations.

Program staff included a physician and psychologist (from the ORFP), the YMCA's program director and nutritionist, and a behavior analyst hired through ORFP. The nutritionist and behavior analyst, working closely with the physician and psychologist, were responsible for primary development and detail of the program format. Program sessions were conducted either by the nutritionist and behavior analyst or by the nutritionist alone.

The HLP was organized to be a part of a continuous program available through the YMCA, beginning with a high-frequency contact period followed by a low-frequency contact period which included standard YMCA offerings (for example, "Slim Living Class," access to exercise facilities, aerobic classes).

Prior to the orientation meeting, lectures were given by ORFP personnel as a part of the YMCA's "Quality of Life" lecture series; notices were placed in local newspapers and the YMCA brochure. A general description of the program and the introduction of the key personnel involved were given at the orientation. Participants signed up for the program at the conclusion of this meeting.

For twenty-six consecutive weeks, meetings were conducted on Wednesday evenings for one-and-a-half hours and on Saturday mornings for one-and-a-half hours. The evening meetings included an interactive lecture on nutrition, a recipe demonstration, and/or methods of food preparation relating to the lesson. The objective was to acquaint participants with the recommended guidelines they needed to follow in order to meet goals of reducing risk factors and living a healthier life-style.

The main emphasis of the evening meetings was on reducing the amount of sugar, fat, and salt in the diet and increasing the amount of complex carbohydrates. The information was presented in such a manner that the participant received a basic understanding of the principles of nutrition. For example, discussed were the chemical structure of a fat and what distinguishes a saturated fat from an unsaturated fat, the physiological reasons for choosing one over the other, and scientific studies to back up these statements. Visual aids and demonstrations were then used to clarify and bring into everyday workable terms the information given in the lecture. Thus, reasons for choosing one food over another were presented, followed by examples and demonstrations that gave the tools with which to go home and use the information.

In addition, at the evening meetings, the behavior analyst led discussions related to the previous week's assignments and experiences. The objectives were to use data collected and other reports by participants to assist them in resolving problems and to determine their course of action for the coming week or a longer time period. Discussions of nontarget performance and of weight loss or gain were discouraged by emphasizing solutions involving the establishment of specific eating patterns and exercise routines. Nutrition and exercise objectives presented by the nutritionist were emphasized. Among other important targets were the development of the group as the primary "helping agents" (rather than the behavior analyst or nutritionist alone), involvement in YMCA or other similar community organizations, family involvement, and interaction with health-related media presentations. During weeks twenty-five and twenty-six, individual sessions with each participant were conducted at which an individual postprogram plan was devised.

The Saturday-morning meetings were used for two main purposes: (a) to provide an exercise class tailored to the needs of the program participants and (b) to provide opportunities for family involvement (either in the exercise or monthly lectures presented by a physician or psychologist). Saturday exercise classes were led by the nutritionist. Participants discussed exercise plans and equipment, took measured/paced walks out-of-doors, and finished with a 10–15 minute warm down which included some floor exercise. Lectures focused on general health issues and were followed by a short discussion period.

Full and partial fitness evaluations were conducted. The full evaluations included bicycle ergometer testing; blood cholesterol, triglycerides, and glucose tests; blood pressure; resting pulse rate; skinfold measures; scale weight; and interviews focusing on health-related concerns, goals, and plans. The partial evaluations included all of the above except the bicycle test and blood work with the exception of the three-month evaluation which included blood work.

Participants were requested to maintain daily records of foods consumed (by time of day). Some recorded amounts and others only types of food. Recording of exercise (type, duration, and pulse rates) was also assigned. A variety of attempts were made to evaluate adherence to techniques presented in the discussions, demonstrations, and so on. Food records, when available, proved most helpful. Records of goal statements and accomplishments, samples of foods prepared at home and brought to meetings, casual discussions of life activities, restaurant visits with participants, and responses to direct verbal probes (for example, did you follow the recommendations from our last meeting?) also were helpful in evaluating adherence.

Outcome Data of the Healthy Life Program

Results from the fitness evaluations and other data sources were discussed at regular Wednesday sessions. Final results were summarized and sent to each participant at the end of the program. Four of the initial fifteen participants dropped out of the program. The remaining eleven participants attended a mean of eighteen Wednesday meetings. Saturday attendance was quite variable across participants. Four attended on twelve or more days, one never attended on Saturday, and the other six averaged six to seven days. Food records were kept for fifteen weeks or more by three participants. The remaining eight averaged six weeks with food records. Exercise data were kept on a sporadic basis, indicating a need for specific contingencies targeted on nutrition recording with this population.

Comparison of initial values with those obtained at six months revealed that all ten participants for whom data were available showed decreases in percent body fat and weight. Percentage decreases in the former ranged between 0.6 and 9.2 (mean = 3.7). Weight loss ranged between 0.5 and 16.0 pounds (mean = 9.9). Blood pressure also showed desired changes for eight participants. Cholesterol levels (total or HDL) decreased in two cases, increased in two cases, and showed no change in four cases (insufficient data were available for the remaining three). Glucose levels were lower for six of the eight participants for whom data were available. Triglyceride levels were lower for five, higher for one, and unchanged for another of the seven participants on whom data were available. On the bicycle test, improvements were noted for seven of the ten individuals. Examination of food records, anecdotal reports, and food demonstrations indicated that at least eight of the participants adjusted their food intake in accordance with the program guidelines.

Follow-up included two dinner engagements (at three and five months post-program) and a fitness evaluation (weighing, skinfold, and bicycle test) at six months. Four participants came to dinner. Three of these had the fitness evaluation. Dinner conversation and ordering patterns were consistent with program guidelines on food consumption and problem-solving strategies.

These preliminary findings are encouraging in that it was possible to obtain several diverse measures of health across a six-month period and decreases in body fat and improved blood pressure and fitness (although slight) were obtained with a rather nonaggressive approach which focused on alternating food composition and moderate excercise rather than restrictive dieting.

Conclusions

We have attempted to provide a general description of what we see as an approximation to a service delivery network, consistent with an integrated-field perspective. This approach, guided by an interbehavioral philosophy, coupled with contemporary scientific knowledge and the hardware necessary to provide concrete data on complex fields, stands in sharp contrast to most contemporary obesity service delivery systems. Many of the latter appear to explain things and events important to obesity and risk-factor management with formulations based upon linear mechanics or indirect measurement. Furthermore, many of these explanations often seem to be influenced primarily by intraverbal functions or other deflections of scientific verbal behavior.

The interdisciplinary characteristic of the approach described here expands the potential impact of the knowledge gained through this endeavor (and its successors). This approach lays the foundation for a holistic understanding necessary for description and intervention in the realm of human behavior. Most certainly, major contributions to such understanding are made by researchers working to isolate specific factors in controlled or simplified contexts (as in the work done on schedules of reinforcement). Just as certainly, major contributions to misunderstanding of human behavior occur when individuals attempt to explain or intervene in complex human affairs armed only with an isolated set of research findings from a simplified setting. When this occurs the inevitable gaps are often filled with myths or other complex conceptual behavior more closely related to special verbal communities than to systematic study of many complex interactions of objects and events over time. The latter is not likely to occur in a setting employing an authentic interdisciplinary, integrated-field approach.

The ORFP and its related programs is a system that is evolving by design. As new information, personnel, and additional disciplines are integrated within the ORFP network, a more complete intervention system and an expanded focus will emerge. Eventually, there may come the time when the knowledge gained from this system will be used to assist others in developing interventions that help individuals avoid obesity or related risk factors altogether and move without interruption along a personal health trajectory.

The authors would like gratefully to acknowledge the contributions of many participants important in the development of this paper: Dr. Dennis J. Delprato for his excellent instruction and feedback with respect to theoretical issues involved in this area; Elizabeth A. Ardito for her contribution to the development of the ORFP and help in editing the paper; Dr. Nan K. Holmes for her continuing contribution to the ORFP; Rena Sutter and Pat Lundy for their help in developing the HLP; Dr. Charles P. Lucas for his pursuit of excellence in obesity research and treatment; and Cheryl Duffy for typing the paper.

References

Ahmad, N., H. Yee, D. Stevenson, S. Taylor, N. Holmes, L. Darga, T. Spafford, and C. Lucas. October 1985. Factors that affect blood pressure reduction with weight loss. Poster presented at the meeting of the joint Conference on Obesity and Non-Insulin Dependent Diabetes, Toronto, Ontario.

Bennett, W., and J. Gurin. 1982. *The dieter's dilemma: Eating less and weighing more.* New York: Basic Books.

Brownell, K. D. 1982. Obesity: Understanding and treating a serious, prevalent, and refactory disorder. *Journal of Consulting and Clinical Psychology* 50:820–40.

Delprato, D. J., and F. D. McGlynn. 1986. Innovations in behavioral medicine. In M. Hersen, R. M. Eisler, and P. M. Miller (Eds.), *Progress in behavior modification*, vol. 20. New York: Academic Press, pp. 67–122.

Fuller, P. R. 1983. *Introductory comments on system science*. Unpublished manuscript.

Franklin, B. A., and J. Scherf. 1985. Personal communication.

Gottman, J. M. 1981. *Time-series analysis: A comprehensive introduction for social scientists*. New York: Cambridge University Press.

Holmes, N. K., E. A. Ardito, D. W. Stevenson, and C. P. Lucas. 1984. Maintenance of weight loss in a heavily overweight population. In J. Storlie and H. A. Jordan (Eds.), *Behavioral Management of Obesity*. Jamaica, N.Y.: Spectrum Publications, 137–150.

Kantor, J. R. 1946. The aims and progress of psychology. *American Scientist* 34: 251–63.

Kantor, J. R. 1953. *The Logic of Modern Science*. Chicago: Principia Press.

Lucas, C. P., D. W. Stevenson, L. Darga, H. Yee, N. Ahmad, N. Holmes, S. Taylor, S. Kasim, and T. Spafford. 1985, November. Change in serum lipids after weight reduction and three and six months of weight maintenance. Paper presented at the meeting of the Central Society for Clinical Research, Chicago, Illinois.

Mackeen, P. C., B. A. Franklin, W. C. Nicholas, and E. R. Buskirk. 1983. Body composition, physical work capacity and physical activity habits at 18 month follow-up of middle-aged women participating in an exercise intervention program. *International Journal of Obesity* 7:61–71.

Mrosovsky, N., and T. L. Powley. 1977. Set points for body weight and fat. *Behavioral Biology* 20: 205–23.

Staddon, J.E.R. 1983. *Adaptive behavior and learning*. Cambridge, England: Cambridge University Press.

Stunkard, A. J. 1975. Presidential address—1974: From explanation to action in psychosomatic medicine: The case of obesity. *Psychosomatic Medicine* 37: 195-236.

Stunkard, A. J., and S. B. Pennick. 1979. Behavior modification in the treatment of obesity: The problem of maintaining weight loss. *Archives of General Psychiatry* 35:801–6.

Taylor, S., D. W. Stevenson, V. Dulmage, and C. P. Lucas. 1985, May. Long-term multimodal, multidisciplinary treatment of obesity and risk factors. Paper presented at the Eleventh Annual Convention of the Association for Behavior Analysis, Columbus, Ohio.

10

Interbehavioral Perspectives on Legal Deviance: Some Considerations of Context

Edward K. Morris, Lisa M. Johnson,
Lynda K. Powell, and James T. Todd

New ideas in therapy are numerous yet troublesome. They are troublesome because therapists have difficulty differentiating new ideas that are important, yet hard to accept, from new ideas that make common sense, yet are spurious. For some therapists, applied behavior analysis and behavior therapy (hereafter, "the behavior therapies") were new ideas that seemed important when introduced, even though slightly unsettling because of a seemingly mechanistic orientation. For other therapists, the behavior therapies seemed spurious from the start because, in part, the approach appeared superficial and unable to get at the heart of the problems being addressed.

This book is based on the assumption that interbehavioral psychology is an important new idea in therapy. The present chapter is a case in point with respect to legal deviance or, more commonly, "crime and delinquency." The chapter, however, takes a slightly different tack: interbehavioral psychology is not simply a new idea in therapy but is, itself, a therapy—a "therapy" for the behavior therapies. Interbehavioral psychology provides therapeutic guidance that meets the challenges of mechanism, spuriousness, and superficiality. In presenting the implications of this perspective for legal deviance, we focus on the predominant contextual features of interbehavioral psychology—interbehavioral history, organismic and environmental setting factors, and the integrated-field perspective as a whole. Before moving to this material, however, let us first provide an

The authors of this chapter are listed alphabetically except for the first. We would like to thank Curtis J. Braukmann and Susan M. Schneider for their comments on earlier versions of the manuscript.

overview of the contextual nature of interbehavioral psychology for legal deviance.

Overview of the Contextual Perspective

To begin with, the term *legal deviance* may seem an unusual one. It is
preferable to "crime and delinquency," however, because it provides a clear
focus on the social nature and definition of a broad set of problems, ranging
from those that most societies find reprehensible most of the time (for example,
murder) to those that some societies find reprehensible only some of the time
(for example, crimes without victims, cf. Schur, 1965). By adopting the term
"legal deviance," we have also sought to avoid labeling individuals, their behavior, and their enviroment as though any one of them possesses some im-
mutable criminal or delinquent property. Moreover, legal deviance suggests the
contextual perspective that is central to the material presented in this chapter.

The contextualism of interbehavioral psychology offers a number of important
perspectives on legal deviance (cf. McKearney, 1977). First, legal deviance
should be seen as a social label that refers to a complex interactive process; it
does not refer to a "thing." Second, legal deviance emerges from a confluence
of multiple, interdependent factors and hence has no inevitable basis or invariable
cause. And third, the structure of legal deviance is variable in its functions and
hence is not comprehensible in terms of its form alone. These characteristics of
the contextual perspective suggest that no one therapy exists for the problem—
there can be no one "vaccine" for crime and delinquency. Much of this chapter
provides specific illustrations of these points.

Legal deviance is ubiquitous. It ranges from frequent, relatively innocuous
crimes without victims to less frequent, but heinous crimes against people.
Combined, the frequency and severity of legal deviance make it a primary public
concern, which has led to numerous and varied attempts to reduce it, ranging
from optimistic measures of prevention and amelioration to the more pessimistic
measures of incapacitation. Among the most optimistic of recent perspectives
has been the behavioral conceptualization of legal deviance within behavioral
sociology (e.g., Burgess & Akers, 1966; Jeffery, 1965) and the application of
the behavioral therapies to legal deviance within behavioral psychology (cf.
Morris, 1980; Nietzel, 1979; for example, Stumphauzer, 1973, 1979). By now
the behavioral literature on legal deviance contains numerous research reports
and texts covering a wide vareity of problems and issues (see Morris, 1978).

Nonetheless, although the behavioral approach to legal deviance has been an
important innovation in all phases of conceptualization and intervention (cf.
Morris & Braukmann, 1987), the approach has not become the panacea some
thought it would be. The reasons for this are many, but they generally fall into
two classses—internal and external. Some of the internal reasons are that some
conceptualizations and applications have been narrow, mechanistic, and superficial (Emery & Marholin, 1977; Geller, Johnson, Hamlin, & Kennedy, 1977).

Among the external reasons for the sometimes limited success of the approach is that society at large, as well as those who develop and implement criminal justice programs (cf. Reppucci & Saunders, 1974), have resisted the approach and misunderstood or misrepresented the implications of a natural science of behavior and its application (Morris, 1985; Todd & Morris, 1983).

J.R. Kantor's interbehavioral psychology (Kantor, 1959), however, offers a broadened and enriched behavioral perspective that begins with the explicit assumption that social problems are complexly and contextually produced and that the fundamental functions of social problems must be addressed rather than their symptoms superficially treated. The interbehavioral perspective also has the positive quality of being compatible with the most experimentally demanding of natural science views on behavior and behavior change (Morris, 1982), as well as offering innovative perspectives for all of the behavioral sciences (see Smith, Mountjoy, & Ruben, 1983). This chapter is not the place to provide an in-depth introduction to interbehavioral psychology; that material may be gleaned from other chapters in this book and from the references cited in the present chapter. Nonetheless, we need to present at least the central characteristics of the approach in order to provide a meaningful context for the material to follow.

At the most fundamental level, the interbehavioral perspective conceptualizes all person-environment interactions, deviant or not, as part of a holistic, interbehavioral field composed of five interacting and mutually interdependent factors: (a) the person (organismic equipment and response forms and functions), (b) the environment (physical dimensions, and stimulus forms and functions), (c) the sensory media through which the organism and environment interact, (d) the organismic and environmental setting factors that function to facilitate or inhibit the stimulus and response functions, and (e) the interbehavioral history through which these functions are initially established.

Many implications can be drawn from this integrated-field orientaion for the analysis of and intervention into legal deviance, but we have chosen to focus on its contextualism, the one characteristic that most clearly avoids mechanism and does not superficially overlook the complexity of person-environment interactions (cf. Sarbin, 1977). In the three sections that follow, we present some implications of the contextual perspective for legal deviance derived from the concepts of interbehavioral history, setting factors, and the integrated field.

Interbehavioral History

Interbehavioral history refers to the past interactions between people and their environments. Interbehavioral history—both phylogenetic and ontogenetic—is the source of the interacting response functions of the person and the stimulus functions of the environment (that is, the functions of a person's behavior and the correlated functions of the environment for that behavior). These interdependent relationships are continually modified by further interactions throughout an individual's lifetime. In a sense, then, interbehavioral history is the context for all current interactions.

Almost every approach to legal deviance acknowledges in some way the role of past history in the determination of behavior. This history, unfortunately, is often transformed into hypothetical, internal mental structures or functions that are said to serve as current and contiguous mediators of the interactions between person and environment. Contextualism rejects such mentalism yet retains the important place of a person's history. In this section of the chapter, we examine three ways in which mentalistic theories circumvent historical causation and illustrate the advantages of the interbehavioral perspective in the explanation of legal deviance in each case. The mentalistic theories on which we focus relate to mental and biological traits or structures, mental and biological processes or functions, and situationism.

Mental and Biological Traits

One form of mentalistic theory explains legal deviance in terms of hypothetical or biological traits or structures that supposedly reside within the individual as the source and cause of deviant interactions. Such biologically based trait theories have become (once again) increasingly popular in the analysis of legal deviance (e.g., Hartl, Monnelley, & Elderkin, 1982; Mednick, 1985; Mednick & Christiansen, 1977, Wilson & Hernstein, 1985). Biological trait theories attempt to explain behavior in terms of the theoretical existence or action of hypothetical biological entities, such as deviance-producing genes, rather than in terms of demonstrated physiological participation. Because these theories depend on hypothetical entities and action, the theories are functionally mentalistic.

Many biological theories of deviance focus on the supposed manifestation of genetic traits. These traits are seen as ever-present structures waiting for the right conditions to release preprogrammed responses or patterns of behavior. Very often, the traits start merely as descriptive categories of observed behavior patterns (e.g., violence), but the terms describing these patterns then become reified as causes of deviance. That is, behavior *described* with trait terminology (e.g., violence) is said to be *caused* by the trait (e.g., by violent "tendencies" or "characteristics"). Once the traits become causes, persons with similar behavior patterns, or who are genetically related to persons with similar behavior patterns, are assumed to possess the same internal trait, whether or not the trait is manifested.

A recent example of a mentalistic genetic trait theory involves the male XYY genotype and its correlation with a larger than average somatotype and low intelligence test score. Numerous studies have reported that a higher proportion of XYY males are found among institutionalized men than in the population at large (e.g, Jacobs, Brunton, Melville, Brittain & McClemont, 1965). These data, in turn, have been taken to support the claim that the XYY genotype is a direct cause of legal deviance through heightened aggressive tendencies (e.g.,

Neilson & Tsuboi, 1969); as it has been put more explicitly: it is "reasonable to assume that antisocial behavior is due to the extra Y chromosome" (Price & Whatmore, 1967, p. 815).

Recent studies and reanalyses of these data, however, have shown that no direct causal relationship exists between the XYY genotype and heightened aggression—the relationship is mediated or conditional on the presence and action of other variables (e.g., physical appearance and body build)—and that the supposition that a greater proportion of XYY males exists in prisons than in the population at large is tenuous (e.g., Pyeritz, Schrier, Madansky, Miller, & Beckwith, 1977). Because many early studies were based on the premise that inner traits, whatever their origin, were the causes of behavior, the histories of the convicted felons were overlooked and few other factors were considered as possible explanations of the correlation. Interbehavioral psychology views genetic and other organismic variables as but one set of factors in a person's historical interaction with the environment. Future research should examine how social processes interact with organismic characteristics (for example, XYY genotype) to shape and maintain deviant behavior, as well as result in differential arrest, prosecution, conviction, and sentencing. We are not questioning the actual physiological and anatomical events that participate in behavior labeled legal deviance; those events clearly warrant investigation in their own right. Physiological reductionism, however, will not provide *the* explanation for this or any other behavior. Behavior is more complex than that.

Mental and Biological Processes

A second form of mentalistic theory explains legal deviance in terms of active mental or biological processes or functions that supposedly intervene between person and environment or between response and stimulus functions. Typically, these active processes are said to mediate (or even actively select and direct) the effect of the environment on the individual's behavior.

An example of such an explanation is S. Yochelson and S.E. Samenow's (1976) proposal that certain forms of legal deviance result, in part, from the mediation of "criminal thinking patterns" that possess a number of dynamic characteristics such as "energy" and "anger." In their description of the role of these thinking patterns, Yochelson and Samenow presented the case of a "criminal" under their treatment who nearly assaulted a mechanic after having had difficulty with car repairs. This individual's behavior was explained in terms of the "metastasis" or "malignant" spread of an angry thinking pattern throughout the thinking process, a mental pehnomenon said not usually to occur in noncriminals.

From an interbehavioral perspective, these criminal thinking patterns are no more than reified constructs or descriptions of correlated covert verbal and emotional activity. As reified hypothetical constructs, the angry thinking patterns are inferred from the deviant behavior itself and are not independently assessed. As correlated activity, neither the verbal nor emotional manifestation of the thinking pattern is explained in terms of any actual functional relations with the person-environment interactions, and neither is the hypothetical causal status of such manifestations established.

An analysis of the interbehavioral history of the person who overreacted to car-repair problems might have revealed the development of stimulus and response functions that resulted in the overreaction and of the anger to which the overreaction was attributed. For example, the man might have previously been successful in achieving his goals through threats and violent activity rather than by more socially acceptable means, such as persuasion and negotiation. Information about this person's interbehavioral history might contribute to the prediction of future legal deviance—prediction that might not be obtained only through inferences about his current "thinking patterns." Furthermore, such information might be used in the development of therapeutic programs for modifying stimulus and response functions so as to alter the future probability of legal deviance. Instead of concentrating on hypothetical, or at best inaccessible and highly intractable internal processes whose causal status is questionable, a therapist might identify the conditions under which people are most likely to become involved in legal deviance and then teach these people to identify those conditions in order to avoid them.

Situationism

An alternative to the mentalistic practice of placing the historical causes of deviance within the person has been to place the causes in the current environment. This alternative is often referred to as "situationism." Situationism, however, can be mentalistic in that the environment, like traits or processes, is treated as though it possessed inherent power to cause or control behavior. From an interbehavioral perspective, situationism, like mentalism, fails to take into account the historically derived functional relationships between individuals and their environments (Knupfer, 1947; Morris, 1982, pp. 208–9).

A good example of the misleading character of situational explanations comes from the work of J.L. Freedman (1975) on crowding and behavior. Common sense, for instance, suggests that crowded living conditions produce crime, and hence crowding is often cited as a situational cause of crime. Indeed, research data show this common sense to be accurate: the crime rate per 100,000 is higher in areas of larger population. A large population, however, as Freedman points out, is not synonymous with a high population density (that is, population per area). When density alone is examined, crowding is only weakly correlated with crime; moreover, crimes of violence are more poorly correlated with density than are crimes against property. In addition, when poverty, educational level, and other demographic characteristics are taken into account no relationship exists between density and crime (Freedman, 1975, pp. 55–69). Indeed, what becomes important in predicting crime is less the situation of crowding per se and more the specific conditions related to architectural residential-commercial functions and the multiple use of the space. In making this argument, we are not asserting that crowding never has deleterious effects—it does, especially in prison settings (Cox, Paulus, & McCain, 1984). Rather, we are pointing out that situational explanations should be analyzed more carefully in terms of the stimulus functions actually involved and their corresponding response functions, both of which are derived through their interactional history.

Put more generally, two of the problems presented by situational explanations are as follows. First, situational accounts have difficulty explaining individual differences in the presence of apparently similar environments—some people emerge from debilitating social conditions with a repertoire of socially appropriate behavior, while others are frequently involved in legal deviance. From the contextualistic perspective, though, apparently similar environments can have vastly different functions for different people depending on the more subtle, but not unpowerful, aspects of their individual interbehavioral histories. The effects of phylogeny aside, the functions of the environment are not inherent within it; the environment acquires its functions as the result of a person's unique interactions with it.

Second, situational accounts do not by themselves explain how certain events acquire or maintain their unique functions for behavior. Correlations of legal deviance with demographic characteristics such as poverty do not shed light on how those correlations came about. An emphasis on interbehavioral history, however, focuses directly on the continuous development and evolution of stimulus and response functions. Information about a person's interbehavioral history can illuminate important causal relationships and point to variables that might be useful in altering behavior. With such knowledge, a therapist could, for example, change those functional relationships responsible for an individual's legal deviance and attempt to modify "situations" that are both statistically and functionally related to legal deviance.

Summary

Approaches to legal deviance that focus on supposed co-temporaneous biological and environmental constructs as explanations of those interactions too often invoke spurious causes on the basis of structural considerations rather than on the basis of functional analyses. Historical causation, however, implicates the continuous process and evolution of person-environment interactions. Moreover, the analysis of person-enviroment interactions in terms of an interbehavioral history of confrontable events suggests concrete steps that can be taken in the description and prediction of legal deviance and in its therapy. Further examples of what some of these steps may be are illustrated by a discussion of setting factors.

Setting Factors

Setting factors are contextual conditions that influence which stimulus-response functions, previously established through an interbehavioral history, will occur at a particular time. More specifically, they facilitate and inhibit previously acquired stimulus and response functions. This "metafunction" of setting factors is itself derived from phylogenetic and ontogenetic contingencies, that is, interbehavioral history. In serving this historically derived function, they are quite distinct from the mentalistic or structural notions of situationism.

Although setting factors are not defined by any formal or structural characteristics, they may be characterized in terms of their locus of action—either organismic or environmental.

Organismic Setting Factors

Organismic setting factors of a *psychological* sort refer to changes in biological conditions within the organism that alter (i.e., facilitate or inhibit) the functions of stimuli and responses of an organism-environment interaction (Kantor, 1947, p. 287). In one sense, of course, a person's organismic equipment (anatomy and physiology) is a setting for all behavior in that it "statically" determines what behaviors a person can or cannot physically perform at a particular moment; this aspect of the organismic equipment is of a *nonpsychological* sort (i.e., of a biological sort). These static determiners may certainly change, both over the lifespan in general and over more circumscribed periods of time. In contrast to organismic setting factors of a nonpsychological sort, which determine what a person can or cannot do, organismic setting factors of a psychological sort "dynamically" influence (facilitate or inhibit) what interactions may or may not occur, that is, what previously established interactions between stimulus and response functions will be present on a particular occasion. For instance, whether or not drugs operate as setting factors of a biological sort to limit or enhance a person's physical capabilities, drugs may also operate as setting factors of a psychological sort to alter the function of the environment for an individual, and vice versa, thereby influencing how the environment is responded to (i.e., drugs may influence a person's perception of reality). Other common examples of organismic setting factors are deprivation and satiation of food or sleep, and illness.

In discussing organismic setting factors with respect to legal deviance, we focus our analysis on one area: the relationship between drugs and legal deviance—especially violence and aggression (cf. Siegal, 1978; Zinberg 1984). In examining drugs as setting factors, we present the implications of a contextual approach with respect to (a) conceptual problems in drug-crime research, (b) the causal status of drugs in violent crime, and (c) the context of current social policy with respect to drug laws.

Conceptual problems in drug-crime research. Perhaps the major conceptual problem in drug-crime research which an interbehavioral perspective might ameliorate is the lack of an overall systematic framework for the research relating drugs to legal deviance (see Roizen & Schneberk, 1977). As with most of psychology, this area of inquiry is composed of many independent theories, each limited in scope.

One of the clearest manifestations of this problem is that research on the interrelationships between drugs and legal deviance often focuses on only one variable at a time. Although this tactic is often a proper one in scientific analysis, it can also lead to (or be the result of) the implicit assumption that single-variable, direct relationships exist between drug-taking and legal deviance (see Greenberg, 1981). In contrast, an interbehavioral perspective argues that no particular factor in an interbehavioral field can be said to have sole causal status—the entire situation must be taken into account (cf. McKearney, 1977). Therapeutic practice, then, should not only focus on treating the drug problem with, for instance, a methadone program, but should also take into account other precipitating factors related to drug abuse (e.g., lack of vocational and social skills) (see Thompson, Koerner, & Grabowski, 1984, for an example of a drug treatment program that does consider such factors).

The causal status of drugs in violent crime. In addition to the problem of the lack of systematization in the drug-crime literature, a conceptual problem relating to the causal status of drugs in violent crimes also exists. For instance, one common assumption about drug use is that drugs are a primary organismic cause of violence and aggression (Siegal, 1978; Szasz, 1974). This logic is seen in the exclusive focus on the pharmacological aspects of drug abuse apparent in many drug laws and drug treatment programs (e.g., methadone treatment). Popular assumptions aside, the facts are that no illicit drug is necessary or sufficient for violent legal deviance (Siegal, 1978; Tinklenberg, 1973).

The many statistical correlations between drug use and violence, of course, cannot be overlooked (see Elliot & Ageton, 1976). The interbehavioral perspective, however, with its emphasis on contextual variables, suggests that drugs, as organismic variables, possess chemical properties, but only behavioral possibilities. Whether or not a drug operates as an organismic setting factor depends not only on the physiological changes it produces from within the organism but also on the person's cultural and individual history and on other aspects of the current environment. Drugs may participate in violent crime, but only in combination with a wide variety of other factors, one of which is the social policy regarding illicit drug use.

Social policy implications. A contextual approach to drug abuse is important not only for examining drug effects on behavior but also for addressing the larger issues of drug use within a social context. In our own culture, the manner in which drug use is regulated (or not) creates a variety of social problems and is not necessarily related to what is actually known about the pharmacological nature of drugs. Two sources of data lend support to this view.

First, drug classification schemes notwithstanding, no strong evidence exists to support distinctions between illicit and licit drugs solely on the basis of their pharmacological effects (Siegal, 1978). For instance, although the Comprehensive Drug Abuse Prevention and Control Act of 1970 classified narcotics and other drugs by "schedules" according to their potential for abuse and current accepted medical usefulness, the classification is not related to the drugs' pharmacological structures, nor does knowledge of the pharmacological structure necessarily allow one to predict that a given drug, out of context, will produce given effects leading to abuse (Jaffe, 1980, p. 576). Moreover, although the approaches taken to control the use of marijuana and heroin are different from those taken toward the use of cigarettes and alcohol, the use of alcohol can certainly be more detrimental than the use of marijuana and, under some circumstances heroin, where even the smallest use of the latter two is defined as "abuse."

Because the pharmacological distinctions among varying classes of drugs are often arbitrary, drug educators and law enforcment officials are seemingly placed in the position of differential "treatment" of drug use on the basis of legalized social sanctions and not on the basis of the ways in which drugs affect behavior. Thus, the problems that drugs cause in a society may be as much a function of social policies related to drug use as they are a function of the drugs those policies seek to regulate (see Stachnik, 1972). Moreover, drug abuse might be more accurately regarded as a symptom of other, more fundamental, social problems rather than as the cause of social problems. In any event, social policies that focused less on drugs themselves and more on the social conditions that promote their use might be more successful in reducing abuse (cf. National Commission on Marijuana and Drug Abuse, 1973).

A second source of data supporting the need to change social policies is the research illustrating that illicit drugs can be used in a responsible and appropriate manner, a fact that is contrary to the implicit assumptions of many current drug policies. L. N. Robins, D. H. Davis, and D. W. Goodwin (1974), for example, have found that Vietnam veterans addicted to narcotics while abroad infrequently remained addicted when they returned to the United States; many veterans were able to use narcotics responsibly or to dispense with them altogether. Other research shows that no necessary relationship exists between the pharmacological effects of drugs and violent crime (cf. Siegal, 1978), which is again contrary to conventional belief. Thus, research suggests that illicit drugs can be used in a manner not harmful to society and, given responsible use, often in a manner not harmful, and sometimes beneficial, to the individual, at least no more harmful than the use of many licit drugs.

Nevertheless, drug abuse is associated with various social problems and hence warrants serious concern and analysis. A contextual perspective of these problems offers some insights different from the usual. For instance, given the present social policies regarding illicit drug use, the maintenance of a heroin habit can be seen as an excellent predictor of membership in a deviant drug culture (see Baridon, 1976). In light of our previous discussion, this membership is partly an artifact of social policies, not of the pharmacological composition of heroin. Ironically, additional and more serious forms of deviance are created in the attempt to suppress drug use. In addition, not only do current drug laws and enforcement policies incur heavy costs on society by fostering deviant subcultures, but the costs of drug law enforcement itself is an additional burden. Other costs include health hazards arising from poor-quality drugs and self-administration, creation of black markets, increases in crime for drug procurement, organized crime, police corruption, and side-effects of arrest and prosecution (for example, job loss) (Stachnik, 1972). These side-effects may be alleviated through a variety of means, for instance, by making drugs less expensive through their availability on a socially controlled basis, as is done with alcohol. Controlled sources of availability could also generate valuable tax revenues which could be applied to the social problems that lead to drug abuse in the first place. In any event, those who develop social policies on drug use should consider the broader social context as a source for their own reactions to drug use, as a source of alternatives for the counterproductive effects those reactions may incur, and as a source for preventative strategies to reduce drug abuse.

Summary. Although drugs can operate as organismic setting factors to affect the probability of legal deviance, that relationship itself does not operate apart from the context of interbehavioral history and other various environmental conditions, the latter to which we now turn.

Environmental Setting Factors

Previously, we described both the static nonpsychological (that is, biological) and dynamic psychological characteristics of organismic setting factors, and we emphasized the latter. Environmental setting factors may likewise be classified and emphasized. Nonpsychological environmental setting factors, that is, the physical structure of the world (e.g., the physical confines of a jail cell), are a static setting for behavior, determining what a person can or cannot do. In contrast, environmental setting factors of a psychological sort function dynamically to affect (i.e., facilitate or inhibit) which stimulus and response functions, established through previous interbehavioral history, may occur at any one time. For instance, the physical confines of a jail cell not only place certain physical limitations on behavior, but may also alter the functions of other people within the cell in ways different from their presence in other environments.

Events that function as environmental setting factors of a psychological sort for legal deviance may be classified as either physical-chemical or social-cultural. A common example of the former is the effect of variations in outdoor lighting on the function of a person targeted for an attempted theft or rape (National Advisory Committee on Criminal Justice Standards and Goals, 1973); what lighting permits one to see or not is a static, nonpsychological setting factor. Examples of social-cultural setting factors of a psychological sort might be the effects of the presence or absence of peers on delinquent activity (Aultman,

1980) or of aversive social interactions on interpersonal violence (Felson & Steadman, 1983; Wahler & Fox, 1981). A particularly good example of aversive social interactions operating as possible setting factors is seen in a study by G. R. Mayer, T. Butterworth, M. Nafpaktitis, and B. Sulzer-Azaroff (1983). These researchers proposed that aversive school environments—both ineffective teacher behavior and poor student performance—might be related to the incidence of school vandalism. By implementing a training package to increase the use of positive reinforcement procedures by teachers and to decrease off-task student behavior, the researchers were successful in improving both teacher and student behavior, and, as a by-product, these effects were accompanied by an 80 percent decrease in school vandalism.

Although a description and classification of the many events and contexts that may operate as setting factors for legal deviance would be useful, that is beyond the scope of the present chapter. Instead, we focus on two broader implications of the setting-factor concept: interdisciplinary research, and therapeutic generalization and maintenance.

Interdisciplinary research. Analyses of environmental setting factors show that the causes of legal deviance cannot be determined independently of their broader context. By including environmental setting factors in such analyses, new areas of research and application are being developed, as exemplified by analyses of the relationship of delinquency to parent-community interactions (e.g., Wahler & Graves, 1983) and family interaction patterns (e.g., Serna, Hazel, Schumaker, & Sheldon, 1984).

Such applied research by itself, however, might not be sufficient for determining all the critical setting factors and might profitably be expanded to include the work of scientists in other disciplines, such as sociologists or social psychologists. A broader, more interdisciplinary perspective may point to research on additional sets of social factors that affect functional relationships within social interactions. These factors may operate directly on a person through, for example, major changes in income and employment (cf. Chester, 1976; Glaser, 1964), educational standing (cf. Burke & Simons, 1965), and marital conflict (cf. Rutter, 1979). These factors may also operate indirectly through the action of similar factors on the behavior of others (e.g., a youth's parents), which may alter, for instance, the context of scheduling of family management practices (cf. Robins & Ratcliff, 1978; Wadsworth, 1979).

As mentioned above, although environmental setting factors of a nonpsychological sort are differentiated from those of a psychological sort, the former are not unimportant in affecting the occurrence of legal deviance and represent a further area for interdisciplinary research that might reduce the need for therapeutic intervention. Strategies stemming from considerations of environmental setting factors of a static, nonpsychological sort might emphasize alterations of the physical settings in which crime occurs, rather than targeting specific individuals (see Harries, 1980; Jeffery, 1971). For example, in urban areas, streets and parks that are isolated, unused, and nonfunctional tend to permit legal deviance, whereas streets and parks designed for multiple use tend to be safer (e.g., Jacobs, 1961). Architectural designs, such as unprotected elevators and stairwells, may also permit legal deviance that might not otherwise occur. The physical design of such environments would seemingly benefit from the joint efforts of professionals from many disciplines, all of whom should be encouraged to contribute.

In summary, scientists within other disciplines have pointed to potentially important setting factors that have been overlooked by therapists. Therapists should be developing procedures for evaluating the importance of these factors and prompting more general descriptive research on the part of others. Therapists and their colleagues in other disciplines could be working together to better effect.

Generalization and maintenance. The second issue to address is the difficulty of attaining generalization and maintenance of therapeutic gains across time, settings, and behaviors in most correctional programs and the implications the interbehavioral perspective offers for this problem.

One set of implications is obvious: the specific programming of environmental setting factors for generalization and maintenance should not be overlooked. Although stimulus events that strengthen and set the occasion for socially effective behavior can be programmed across settings and time, these events may not have these functions outside of relevant setting factors. Interventions that seek to promote generalization and maintenance, but that simply focus on programming specific social stimuli and responses, are not likely to succeed. Those interventions must also program the setting factors that establish the effectiveness (or lack thereof) of these stimuli and responses if long-lasting change is to be produced.

Families of delinquents, for example, often display interaction patterns that act as setting factors incompatible with establishing positive and effective relationships among their members. These families display multiple schedules of aversive control, misapply schedules of reinforcement and punishment, and lack parental monitoring of childrens' whereabouts, household rules, and problem-solving skills (Patterson, 1982). Such setting factors must be taken into account when programming for generalization and maintenance.

Another setting factor that might be considered in this regard is the context of reinforcement. For instance, with respect to the "matching law" (see Epling & Pierce, 1983), the effectiveness of reinforcement from one source (for example, family members) is contextually dependent on rates of reinforcement from other sources (for example, peer groups) and vice versa. Any increase in the rate of reinforcement from sources that are not the target of intervention would, everything being equal, decrease the effectiveness of "therapeutic" reinforcement. Thus, when programming for generalization, the therapist should be sensitive to rates of reinforcement being obtained by clients from other sources. In addition, therapists might also attend to such setting factors as the quantitative and qualitative properties of behavior-environment interactions. For instance, the effects of some attempts at generalization may depend on such factors as the rate of behavior and various schedule characteristics (cf. Morse & Kelleher, 1977).

Another set of implications of the setting-factor concept for generalization and maintenance is that research in this area needs an organized conceptual framework. The literature on generalization and maintenance generally describes various strategies drawn from successful pratice (e.g., Stokes & Baer, 1977) but rarely ties these practices to an overall conceptual analysis of the issues involved. Although specific techniques may be quite useful (e.g., Fowler & Baer, 1981), when they fail few other conceptually guided directions are immediately obvious.

A conceptualization of generalization and maintenance in terms of differences and similarities among setting factors, as well as other aspects of the interbehavioral field, might usefully supplement the technology at hand. This approach is compatible with some recent arguments for the analysis of generalization in terms of stimulus-control processes (e.g., Kirby, Bickel, & Holburn, 1983; cf. Bickel & Etzel, 1985). Although many techniques for promoting generalization are already compatible with a stimulus-control perspective (for example, programming common stimuli), the conceptual analysis of generalization lags behind. For instance, generalization is still too often conceptualized as a hypothetical process, perhaps even organismic in nature, rather than as the specific outcome of certain relationships accruing from past organism-environment interactions (cf. Stevenson & Hemingway, 1984). At the very least, a stimulus-control conceptualization is more positive and specific than analyses couched in terms of the presence or absence of some vague process of generalization. We suggest, then, that by developing an approach to generalization and maintenance based on an integrated conceptual system, the probability is increased that the generalization-promoting behavior of therapists will generalize to new problems when old techniques fail.

Summary. The concept of the environmental setting factor is the complementary adjunct to organismic setting factors, and between them they make clear that all causes have contexts. Neither set of factors, however, functions apart from the general integrated-field characteristic of interbehavioral psychology, to which we turn for the final section of the chapter.

The Integrated-Field Perspective

Interbehavioral psychology offers an integrated-field or systems perspective that is holistic in nature; that assumes strong, dynamic, reciprocal interactions among the participating factors; and that emphasizes the continuous nature of person-environment interactions. The interbehavioral perspective rejects the traditional undirectional explanation of causation, as well as the assumption that causation can be reduced to the action of any single discrete causal agent or event. Psychological interactions include the entire field of participating organismic and environmental events, which are interdependent and thus interrelated. This interrelatedness is described as comprising a system (Kantor, 1950).

In this section, we focus on family interaction processes as an example of a predominant system of which delinquent youths are a part. In doing so, we discuss three specific implications of the interbehavioral perspective in this area: the conceptualization of family interactions as a system, research investigating the social interaction systems of families of delinquents, and therapeutic intervention into famly interactions from a systems perspective.

Family Interactions as a System

By conceptualizing family interactions as a system, the focus of research and intervention moves from simply examining how the behavior of one person affects that of another, to an examination of functional interrelationships or patterns among the behaviors of all family members. Given that certain family interaction patterns can be related to such problems as legal deviance, researchers should focus their efforts in three ways. First, they should identify recurrent sequences of interactions that characterize families with children and adolescents who engage in excessive legal deviance and that differentiate such families from those without such problems. Second, they should then specify those interaction patterns that are most closely tied to the occurrence of specific legal deviance. And third, they should devise intervention strategies appropriate for the family system in question. By viewing family interactions as a system of organized patterns and recurrent sequences, rather than as a collection of unidirectional, or even bidirectional, influences, a more realistic, complete, and accurate picture of family problems can be obtained.

Research Methods for Analyzing Systems

The concept of patterning in family interactions leads to a second implication: therapists who examine such processes should employ research methods that retain the naturally occurring order of events and the reciprocal nature of the interactions (Gottman & Notarius, 1978; Lichtenberg & Powell, 1984). The raw materials for studying family interaction patterns are the interactive relationships as they occur in nature. Often, however, the ordering of these events is lost when data are converted into various forms for analysis, especially when summary data obscure important functional relationships. Moreover, many research methods employ unidirectional analyses in which the influence of parents on their children is studied in isolation from the effects of the children on their parents. For example, most socialization research has focused solely on the effects of parent behavior (e.g., father-absence, cf. Jurich, 1979), and not also on child effects (Bell & Harper, 1977). In addition, although applied research from a ''child effects'' perspective has examined how youths affect their interactions with teachers (e.g., Polirstok & Greer, 1977), police officers (e.g., Werner, Minkin, Minkin, Fixsen,

Phillips, & Wolf, 1975), and parents (e.g., Kifer, Lewis, Green, & Phillips, 1974), this research also retains a one-way direction of focus, albeit in a different direction, that does not identify reciprocal influences.

Unfortunately, most research designs, whether within- or between-subjects, do not allow reciprocal effects to be detected. The designs and their attendant methods of analysis "segment" the ongoing sequences of events that constitute the dysfunctional system such that the pattern of the interacting functional relationships is obscured. In order to retain the interlocking, reciprocal nature of these interactions, alternative methods of analysis need to be employed. Among the appropriate methods currently available are Markov chain analyses (Suppeys & Atkinson, 1960), lag sequential analyses (Sackett, 1979), and information theory analyses (Attneave, 1959)—all of which are derived conceptually from conditional sequential dependencies among events occurring over time.

Some researchers have attempted to identify recurrent behavior patterns within interactional sequences, but progress has been constrained by the limitations of the methodologies typically employed. Nonetheless, researchers have found that families with adolescent delinquents evidence distinctly different patterns than families with adolescents having no identified problems. For instance, in problem-solving tasks, families with delinquents have more silent periods, convey less information, and agree less often than families with no delinquents (e.g., Haley, 1964; Ferreira & Winter, 1965; Ferreira, Winter, & Poindexter, 1966; Patterson, 1982). This research suggests that family interaction patterns can be identified and that specific behavior patterns may, in fact, describe families with delinquent adolescents. This research, however, has focused only on describing family interaction patterns, not on intervening into them.

Intervention into Family Systems

By taking an interbehavioral approach to family interaction patterns, each of the factors in the interbehavioral field, as well as the specific variables comprising each factor, can be identified as possible contributors to the development and maintenance of delinquency. Identifying these factors and their specific contributions provides some suggestions for where to intervene in order to produce effective and long-lasting change. In the family process research conducted to date, the assumption is often made that intervening in these identified factors will have a direct effect on legal deviance. Except for the work of Patterson (e.g., Patterson, 1982) and Alexander (e.g., Alexander & Parsons, 1973), however, few attempts have been made to translate the results of the earlier descriptive research into actual intervention strategies. In addition, even when interventions are effective in altering family interaction patterns, the link to reductions in legal deviance is not always clear. In contrast, Patterson's and Alexander's research, which intervenes into family processes by teaching parenting and communication skills, points to the fruitfulness of integrating intervention programs with field-descriptive analyses of the multiple interactive factors in a family system.

Conclusion

We have attempted to be specific in this chapter about the implications of the contextual nature of interbehavioral psychology for legal deviance, but let us conclude more generally. Perhaps the most fundamental point of this chapter is that the narrow focus on individuals, or even small groups, outside of the contexts through which their legal deviance is developed and maintained, will often not be conducive for effecting long-lasting change. Legal deviance is a problem as large as society itself and should be approached and analyzed as such. New ideas in therapy can become part of the problem rather than part of the solution when they focus on individual elements in the social system and not on the system itself (cf. Holland, 1978). Practical means of altering large-scale social systems are, of course, beyond the capabilities of individual therapists, but a contextual or systems perspective—even if constrained by the practicalities of the moment— will be more effective than no contextual perspective at all. The natural science of behavior will continue to evolve in comprehensiveness, conceptual adequacy, and effectiveness as it moves away from mechanism and toward contextualism and the integrated-field perspective. From the latter, we believe, will come innovative therapeutic practices. The effects of these practices, however, can only be determined if the practices are implemented. That is the task at hand.

Perhaps by having described and illustrated the value of the contextual perspective in this chapter, the narrow, mechanistic, and superficial use of various therapeutic programs can be reduced and improved therapeutic programs set as an attainable goal for today. The ideal of solving the large-scale social problem of legal deviance from a contextual perspective can serve as a superordinate goal for tomorrow.

References

Alexander, J. F., and B. V. Parsons. 1973. Short-term behavioral intervention with delinquent families: Impact on family process and recidivism. *Journal of Abnormal Psychology* 81: 219–23.

Attneave, F. 1959. *Application of information theory to psychology*. New York: Holt.

Aultman, M.G. 1980. Group involvement in delinquents: A study of offense types and male-famale participation. *Criminal Justice and Behavior* 7:185–92.

Baridon, P. C. 1976. *Addiction, crime, and social policy*. Lexington, Mass.: Lexington Books.

Bell, R. Q., and L. V. Harper (Eds.) 1977. *Child effects on adults*. Hillsdale, N.J.: Lawrence Erlbaum Associates.

Bickel, W. K., and B. C. Etzel. 1985. The quantal nature of controlling stimulus-response relations as measured in tests of stimulus generalization. *Journal of the Experimental Analysis of Behavior* 44:245–70.

Burgess, R. L., and R. L. Akers. 1966. A differential association-reinforcement theory of criminal behavior. *Social Problems* 14:128–47.

Burke, N. S., and A. E. Simons. 1965, March. Factors which precipitate dropouts and delinquency. *Federal Probation,* pp. 28–32.

Chester, C. R. 1976. Relative deprivation as a cause of property crime. *Crime and Delinquency* 22:17–30.

Cox, V. C., P. B. Paulus, and G. McCain. 1984. Prison crowding research: The relevance of prison housing standards and a general approach regarding crowding phenomena. *American Psychologist* 39:1148–1460.

Elliott, D. S., and A. R. Ageton. 1976. The relationship between drug use and crime among adolescents. In Research Triangle Institute, *Appendix to drug use and crime: Report of the panel on drug use and criminal behavior.* Springfield, Va.: National Technological Information Service, NTIS No. PB259 167, pp. 297–322.

Emery, R. E., and D. Marholin. 1977. An applied behavior analysis of delinquency. *American Psychologist* 32:860–73.

Epling, F. W., and D. W. Pierce. 1983. Applied behavior analysis: New directions from the laboratory. *The Behavior Analyst* 6:27–37.

Felson, R. B., and H. J. Steadman. 1983. Situation factors in disputes leading to criminal violence. *Criminology* 21:59–74.

Ferreira, A. J., and W. D. Winter. 1965. Family interaction and decision-making. *Archives of General Psychiatry* 13:214–23.

Ferreira, A. J., W. D. Winter, and E. J. Poindexter. 1966. Some interactional variables in normal and abnormal families. *Family Process* 5:60–75.

Fowler, S., and D. M. Baer. 1981. "Do I have to be good all day?" The timing of delayed reinforcement as a factor in generalization. *Journal of Applied Behavior Analysis* 14:13–24.

Freedman, J. L. 1975. *Crowding and behavior.* New York: Viking Press.

Geller, E. S., D. F. Johnson, P. H. Hamlin, and T. D. Kennedy. 1977. Behavior modification in prison: Issues, problems, and compromises. *Criminal Justice and Behavior* 4:11–43.

Glaser, D. 1964. *The effectiveness of a prison and parole system.* Indianapolis: Bobbs-Merrill.

Gottman, J. M. and C. Notarius. 1978. Sequential analysis of observation data using Markov chains. In T. Kratochwill (Ed.), *Single subject research: Strategies for evaluating change.* New York: Academic Press, pp. 237–85.

Greenburg, S. W. 1981. Alcohol and crime: A methodological critique of the literature. In J. J. Collins (Ed.), *Drinking and crime: Perspectives on the relationships between alcohol consumption and criminal behavior.* New York: Guilford Press, pp. 70–109.

Haley, J. 1964. Research on family patterns: An instrument survey. *Family Process* 3:41–65.

Harries, K. D. 1980. *Crime and the environment.* Springfield, Ill.: Charles C. Thomas.

Hartl, E. M, E. P. Monnelly, and R. D. Elderkin. 1982. *Physique and delinquent behavior.* New York: Academic Press.

Holland, J. G. 1978. Behaviorism: Part of the problem or part of the solution? *Journal of Applied Behavior Analysis* 11:163–74.

Jacobs, J. 1961. *The death and life of great American cities.* New York: Random House.

Jacobs, P. A., M. Brunton, M. M. Melville, R. P. Brittain, and W. F. McClemont. 1965. Aggressive behavior, mental subnormality, and the XYY male. *Nature* 213:815.

Jaffe, J. H. 1980. Drug addiction and drug abuse. In A. G. Gilman, L. S. Goodman, and A. Gilman (Eds.), *The pharmacological basis of therapeutics*. New York: Macmillan, pp. 535–84.

Jeffery, C. R. 1965. Criminal behavior and learning theory. *Journal of Criminal Law, Criminology, and Police Science* 56:294–300.

Jeffery, C. R. 1971. *Crime prevention through environmental design*. Beverly Hills, Calif.: Sage.

Jurich, A. P. 1979. Parenting adolescents. *Family Perspective* 13:137–49.

Kantor, J. R. 1947. *Problems in physiological psychology*. Granville, Ohio: Principia Press.

Kantor, J. R. 1950. *Psychology and logic*, vol. 2. Chicago: Principia Press.

Kantor, J. R. 1959. *Interbehavioral psychology*. Granville, Ohio: Principia Press.

Kifer, R. E., M. A. Lewis, D. R. Green, and E. L. Phillilps. 1974. Training predelinquent youths and their parents to negotiate conflict situations. *Journal of Applied Behavior Analysis* 7:357–64.

Kirby, K. C., W. K. Bickel, and S. W. Holburn. 1983, May. *Toward an explicit science of generalization: A stimulus-control interpretation*. Paper presented at the meeting of the Association for Behavior Analysis, Milwaukee, Wisconsin.

Knupfer, G. 1947. Portrait of an underdog. *Public Opinion Quarterly* 11:103–14.

Lichtenberg, J. W., and L. K. Powell. 1984, May. *Methods of sequential analysis for studying family interactions*. Paper presented at the meeting of the Association for Behavior Analysis, Nashville, Tennessee.

McKearney, J. W. 1977. Asking questions about behavior. *Perspectives in Biology and Medicine* 21:109–19.

Mayer, G. R., T. Butterworth, M. Nafpaktitis, and B. Sulzer-Azaroff. 1983. Preventing school vandalism and improving discipline: A three year study. *Journal of Applied Behavior Analysis* 16:355–69.

Mednick, S. 1985. Crime in the family tree. *Psychology Today* 19 (3): 58–61.

Mednick, S., and K. O. Christiansen. 1977. *Biosocial bases of criminal behavior*. New York: Wiley.

Michael, J. 1982. Distinguishing between discriminative and motivational functions of stimuli. *Journal of the Experimental Analysis of Behavior* 37:149–55.

Morris, E. K. 1978. A brief review of legal deviance: References in behavior analysis and delinquency. In D. Marholin (Ed.), *Child behavior therapy*. New York: Gardner Press, pp. 214–38.

Morris, E. K. 1980. Applied behavior analysis for criminal justice practice: Some current dimensions. *Criminal Justice and Behavior* 7:131–45.

Morris, E. K. 1982. Some relationships between interbehavioral psychology and radical behaviorism. *Behaviorism* 10:187–216.

Morris, E. K. 1985. Public information, dissemination, and behavior analysis. *The Behavior Analyst* 8:95–110.

Morris, E. K., and C. J. Braukmann. (Eds). 1987. *Behavioral approaches to crime and delinquency: Application, research, and theory*. New York: Plenum.

Morse, W. H., and R. T. Kelleher. 1977. Determinants of reinforcement and punishment. In W. K. Honig and J.E.R. Staddon (Eds.), *Handbook of operant behavior*. Englewood Cliffs, N.J.: Prentice-Hall, pp. 174–200.

National Advisory Commission on Criminal Justice Standards and Goals. 1973. *Corrections*. Washington, D.C.: U.S. Government Printing Office.

National Commission on Marijuana and Drug Abuse. 1973. *Drug use in America: Problem in perspective*. Washington, D.C.: U.S. Government Printing Office.

Neilson, J., and T. Tsuboi. 1969. Intelligence, EEG, personality deviation and criminality in patients with XYY syndrome. *British Journal of Psychiatry* 115:965.

Nietzel, M. T. 1979. *Crime and its modification: A social learning perspective*. Elmsford, N.Y.: Pergamon Press.

Patterson, G. R. 1982. *Coercive family processes*. Champaign, Ill.: Research Press.

Polirstok, S. R., and P. D. Greer. 1977. Remediation of mutually aversive interactions between a problem student and four teachers by training the student in reinforcement techniques. *Journal of Applied Behavior Analysis* 10:707–16.

Price, W. H., and P. B. Whatmore. 1967. Criminal behavior and the XYY male. *Nature* 208:1351–52.

Pyeritz, R., H. Schreir, C. Madansky, L. Miller, and J. Beckwith. 1977. The XYY male: The making of a myth. In Ann Arbor Science for the People Editorial Collective (Eds.), *Biology as a social weapon*. Minneapolis: Burgess, pp. 86–100.

Reppucci, N. D., and T. J. Saunders. 1974. Social psychology of behavior modification: Problems of implementation in natural settings. *American Psychologist* 29–649–60.

Robins, A., and K. S. Ratcliff. 1978. Risk factors in the continuation of childhood antisocial behavior into adulthood. *International Journal of Mental Health* 7:96–116.

Robins, L. N., D. H. Davis, and D. W. Goodwin. 1974. Drug use by U.S. Army enlisted men in Vietnam: A follow-up on their return home. *American Journal of Epidemiology* 99:235–49.

Roizen, J., and D. Schneberk. 1977. Alcohol and crime. In M. Aarens, T. Cameron, J. Roizen, R. Room, D. Schneberk, and D. Wingard (Eds.) *Alcohol, casualties, and crime*. Berkeley, Calif.: Social Research Group, pp. 289–465.

Rutter, M. 1979. Protective factors in children's responses to stress and disadvantage. In M. Kent and J. E. Rolf (Eds.), *Primary prevention and psychopathology: Social competence in children*, vol. 3. Hanover, N.H.: University Press of New England.

Sackett, G. 1979. The lag sequential analysis of contingency and cyclicity in behavioral interaction research. In J. Osofsky (Ed.), *Handbook of infant development*. New York: Wiley, pp. 623–49.

Sarbin, T. R. 1977. Contextualism: A world view for modern psychology. In A. W. Langfield (Ed.), *Nebraska Symposium on Motivation*, vol. 24. Lincoln: University of Nebraska Press, pp. 1–41.

Schnelle, J. F., R. E. Kirchner, J. W. Macrae, M. P. McNees, R. H. Eck, S. Snodgrass, J. D. Casey, and P. H. Uselton. 1978. Police evaluation research: An experimental and cost-benefit analysis of a helicopter patrol in a high crime area. *Journal of Applied Behavior Analysis* 11:121.

Schur, E. M. 1965. *Crimes without victims*. Englewood Cliffs, N.J.: Prentice-Hall.

Serna, L. A., S. Hazel, J. B. Schumaker, and J. Sheldon. 1984, May. *Teaching reciprocal skills to parents and their delinquent adolescents*. Paper presented at the meeting of the Association of Behavior Analysis, Nashville, Tennesse.

Siegal, R. K. 1978. Phencyclidine, criminal behavior, and the defense of diminished capacity. In R. C. Peterson and R. C. Stillman (Eds.), *PCP—Phencyclidine abuse: An appraisal.* Rockville, Md.: National Institute on Drug Abuse, DHEW Publication No. 21, pp. 272–88.

Smith, N. W., P. T. Mountjoy, and D. H. Ruben. (Eds). 1983. *Reassessment in psychology: The interbehavioral alternative.* Washington, D.C.: University Press of America.

Stachnik, T. J. 1972. The case against criminal penalties for illicit drug use. *American Psychologist* 27:637–42.

Stevenson, D. W., and M. J. Hemingway. 1984. Abstraction vs. confrontation. *The Interbehaviorist* 13:7–8.

Stokes, T. F., and D. M. Baer. 1977. An implicit technology of generalization. *Journal of Applied Behavior Analysis* 10:349–67.

Stumphauzer, J. S. (Ed.). 1973. *Behavior modification with delinquents.* Springfield, Ill.: Charles C. Thomas.

Stumphauzer, J. S. (Ed.). 1979. *Progress in behavior modification with delinquents.* Springfield, Ill.: Charles C. Thomas.

Suppeys, P., and R. V. Atkinson. 1960. *Markov learning models for multiperson interactions.* Stanford, Calif.: Stanford Press.

Szasz, T. 1974. *Ceremonial chemistry: The ritual persecution of drugs, addicts, and pushers.* New York: Anchor Press/Doubleday.

Thompson T., J. Koerner, and J. Grabowski. 1984. Brokerage model rehabilitation for opiate dependence: A behavioral analysis. In J. Grabowski, M. L. Stitzer, and J. E. Henningfield (Eds.), *Behavioral techniques in drug abuse treatment.* Rockville, Md.: National Institute on Drug Abuse. DHHS Publication No. ADM 84–1282; Research Monograph 46, pp. 131–46.

Tinklenberg, J. R. 1973. Alcohol and violence. In P. Bourne and R. Fox (Eds.), *Alcoholism: Progress in research and treatment.* New York: Academic Press, pp. 195–210.

Todd, J. T., and E. K. Morris. 1983. Misconception and miseducation: Presentations of radical behaviorism in psychology textbooks. *The Behavior Analyst*, 6:153–60.

Wadsworth, M. 1979. *Roots and delinquency: Infancy, adolescence, and crime.* New York: Barnes & Noble.

Wahler, R. G., and J. J. Fox. 1981. Setting events in applied behavior analysis: Toward a conceptual and methodological expansion. *Journal of Applied Behavior Analysis* 14:322–38.

Wahler, R. G., and M. G. Graves. 1983. Setting events in social networks: Ally or enemy in child behavior therapy? *Behavior Therapy* 14:19–36.

Werner, J. S., N. Minkin, B. L. Minkin, D. R. Fixsen, E. L. Phillips, and M. M. Wolf. 1975. Intervention package: An analysis to prepare juvenile delinquents for encounters with police officers. *Criminal Justice and Behavior* 2:55–84.

Wilson, J. Q., and R. J. Herrnstein. 1985. *Crime and human nature.* New York: Simon and Schuster.

Yochelson, S., and S. E. Samenow. 1976. *The criminal personality. Volume I: A profile for change.* New York: Jason Aronson.

Zinberg, N. E. 1984. *Drug, set, and setting: The basis for controlled intoxicant use.* New Haven, Conn.: Yale University Press.

11

An Interbehavioral Perspective on Parent Training for Families of Developmentally Delayed Children

Lynne A. Daurelle, James J. Fox, William E. MacLean, Jr., and Ann P. Kaiser

Behavioral parent training refers to inverventions based on social learning principles that teach parents to train their own child. Behavioral parent training has been used successfully to treat virtually every type of childhood behavior disorder such as toilet training (Butler, 1976), tantrum behavior (Williams, 1959), noncompliance (Forehand, Sturgis, McMahon, Aguar, Green, Wells, & Breiner, 1979), autism (Lovaas, Koegel, Simmons, & Long, 1973), as well as a variety of everyday problems such as whining, squabbles between siblings, and mealtime problems (Barnard, Christopherson, & Wolf, 1977). Interventions are typically directed toward the referred child, although some programs have included the entire family.

Although behavioral parent-training programs for families of handicapped children frequently yield positive outcomes (see reviews by Baker, 1976; Snell & Beckman-Brinkley, 1984), they are not uniformly effective (e.g., Baker, Heifetz, & Murphy, 1980). It is the contention of some authors that these failures have been the result of the insufficiency of the model upon which most behavioral parent-training programs are based (Daurelle & Fox, 1984; Wahler, 1980; Wahler & Fox, 1981).

The purpose of this chapter is to analyze the current literature on behavioral parent training with developmentally delayed children and to propose an expansion of the prevailing framework used in working with these families. It is proposed that the incorporation of J. R. Kantor's (1959) interbehavioral frame-

Preparation of this manuscript was supported in part by a research assistantship at the Child Study Center at Peabody College and by three grants from NICHD: HD15051, IMRID 630426, and MR 630367.

work into the "three-term contingency" would increase the effectiveness and durability of our intervention efforts.

In order to examine the current status of behavioral parent-training methods with families of developmentally delayed children, it will be helpful to begin with a discussion of the theoretical underpinnings of the three-term contingency.

Background

The Three-Term Contingency and Clinical Intervention

The three-term contingency is B. F. Skinner's (1953, 1974) conceptual unit of analysis. Its component parts include "the antecedent eliciting (S^E) and/or discriminative (S^D) stimuli, respondent (R^R) and/or operant (R_O) behavior, and consequent reinforcing stimuli (S^R). Although the issue of temporality in the sequence of these component parts is not explicitly discussed, most practitioners appear to agree with Guthrie (1935) in their insistence upon immediate contiguity between each part. Although Skinner (1953) is quite clear that the organism is constantly immersed in, and is part of, the environment, researchers in the experimental analysis of behavior, for the most part, have taken single variables as the subject of investigation.

The three-term contingency, along with several other social learning constructs, such as modeling and imitation (Bandura, 1969), has been the basis of many clinical intervention techniques. Most behavioral interventions have been conducted in clinic settings, although there was early recognition that treatment in the natural environment, such as home, school, or job, could lead to more durable, generalized effects (Tharp & Wetzel, 1969). In the case of an intervention program targeting children, emphasis upon treatment in the natural environment would clearly lead to a recognition of the need to work with the child's parents.

Behavioral Parent Training

Behavioral parent training is a triadic, as opposed to dyadic, intervention model (Tharp & Wetzel, 1969). That is, the parent trainer or therapist teaches the parent, who in turn trains the child. The parent is taught behavioral principles in order to change specific child behaviors. In a typical parent-training program, the parent trainer presents the parent with a prepackaged program consisting of a predetermined number of training sessions (Lutzker, McGimsey, McRae, & Campbell, 1983). The next step is to have the parent or an independent observer collect data on targeted parent and child behaviors to ascertain whether change is occurring.

The most important assumptions of behavioral parent training are that (a) child problem behaviours are largely a function of inappropriate or misapplied parent-dispensed contingencies, (b) parents can be taught to rearrange these contingencies to increase appropriate child behavior and teach adaptive skills, and (c) the resulting child behavior change will, in turn, reinforce and maintain parents' continued use of these procedures (Daurelle & Fox, 1984).

Behavioral parent training itself is a relatively recent mode of intervention. The first paper demonstrating the use of behavior modification techniques with the parent as therapist was published by C. Williams (1959), and it was not until the mid–1960s that the use of parents as behavior change agents began to gain wide acceptance. In these early studies, parents were involved minimally in the program, as they simply carried out instructions under the supervision of a trainer on a single problem behavior (e.g., Straughan, 1964; Williams, 1959). Following these early studies, parents were involved to a greater extent (Russo, 1964; Sloane, Johnston, & Bijou, 1967), and parent training shifted from the clinic to the home as more complex behavior problems were targeted for treatment (Hawkins, Peterson, Schweid, & Bijou, 1966; Risley, 1968). More recently, parents have been included in the formation of treatment goals, changing the focus of the parent as "behavioral technician" to the parent as "behavioral engineer" (Baker, Heifetz, & Murphy, 1980; Patterson, 1971; Wahler & Graves, 1983). Modes of training have included didactic instructions, modeling, assigned readings, direct coaching, programmed materials, group discussion, videotapes, and textbooks. Parents have been trained in groups (Adesso & Lipson, 1981; Glogower & Sloop, 1976) and individually (Baum & Forehand, 1981; Mira, 1970). Training approaches usually depend upon the severity and complexity of the child's presenting problem.

The majority of behavioral parent-training interventions concentrate solely on the mother-child dyadic interactions to the exclusion of the rest of the family members and the surrounding social networks (Snell & Beckman-Brinkley, 1984). In many cases this exclusive focus on dyadic interchange has proven adequate in producing positive change in child behavior (see Berkowitz & Graziano, 1972; Johnson & Katz, 1973; O'Dell, 1974). However, there is a growing body of evidence to suggest that extradyadic factors can influence behavioral parent-training outcome.

Extradyadic variables that have been implicated in the outcome of behavioral parent training include maternal depression (Griest, Wells, & Forehand, 1979), socioeconomic status (Clark & Baker, 1983; Rose, 1974a), parent education level (Clark, Baker, & Heifetz, 1982), previous parent training or counseling experience (Baker, 1976), parent insularity (Wahler, 1980; Wahler & Afton, 1980), major disruptive events (Baker, 1980), parental adjustment (Griest & Forehand, 1982), and marital problems (Johnson & Lobitz, 1974; Oltmanns, Broderick, & O'Leary, 1977; Reisinger, Frangia, & Hoffman, 1976).

When one considers the extra stressors that are usually present in families of developmentally disabled children (Friedrich & Friedrich, 1981), extradyadic factors become even more influential in the effectiveness of an intervention program. This influence of extradyadic factors has particular implications for behavioral parent training in families with a developmentally delayed child.

The Impact of a Handicapped Child on the Family

Clearly, family functioning is influenced by the presence of a handicapped child (Farber & Ryckman, 1965). Disruptions in family functioning usually occur for some period of time following the identification of the child's handicap (Davis, 1967; Farber, 1968) and in some cases the disruption may continue indefinitely. The disruption may lead to a higher than average divorce and desertion rate (Bergreen, 1971; Tew, Laurence, Payne, & Rawnsley, 1977), increased social isolation (McAllister, Butler, & Lei, 1973), increased marital difficulties (Fowle, 1968; Freidrich & Friedrich, 1981), decreased family leisure time (DeMyer & Goldberg, 1983), parental depression (Burden, 1980), parent emotional difficulties (Cummings, Bayley, & Rie, 1966; Farber, 1959) and sibling adjustment problems (Grossman, 1972; Poznanski, 1969).

In a review of the literature on family adaptation to a handicapped child, R. Jeffries (1983) described specific variables that appear to mediate family adjustment to the child. These include type/severity of handicap, family resources and environmental circumstances, early attachment between parent and child, parental characteristics, family size and child's birth order, and child's gender.

It follows, then, that the multiplicity of factors that affect family adjustment warrants a more complex intervention than is currently available. One such approach that accommodates a multiplicity of factors in a family system is that of Kantor (1959).

Kantor's Interbehaviorism

Kantor's (1966) conception of an interbehavioral psychology proposes that behavior occurs within a field that consists of the action of the organism, the action of the stimulus, the setting factors, the media of contact, and the interbehavioral history.

A particularly interesting component of the interbehavioral field is the concept of setting factors. Kantor noted that

in a general way the setting factors of interbehavioral fields operate to give pattern and distinction to the specific behavior segments in which they are components. They also serve to facilitate the occurrence of the particular response-stimulus coordinations or to inhibit their performance. (1966, p. 387).

Setting factors, or setting events as some have labeled them (Bijou & Baer, 1961), can include *internal* organismic or biological conditions and *external* environmental conditions (both physical-chemical and social-cultural). Setting events are differentiated from discriminative stimuli by the complexity of the behavioral environmental event, the temporal proximity of the event to the occurrence of behavior, and the effect of the event on behavioral performance. Some authors consider the setting event to be distinct from the three-term contingency, while others (Leigland, 1984; Michael, 1982) claim the concept is too broad and ill-defined for usage in as highly precise a discipline as behavioral psychology (Brown, Bryson-Brockmann, & Fox, 1984). In defense of the concept, R. G. Wahler and his colleagues have provided considerable evidence that the setting-event concept can be useful in describing and predicting previously perplexing phenomena that were "too temporally removed, environmentally complex, [or] non-reinforcement linked to be classified as discriminative stimuli" (Wahler & Hann, in press, p. 13).

Comparison of Interbehavioral Psychology with Existing Theoretical Frameworks

The frameworks of Kantor and Skinner have much in common; the disagreement appears to be in the unit of analysis. By allowing consideration of events that are temporally removed and environmentally complex, Kantor's setting-event concept permits an analysis of more *molar* units of behavior than has been traditionally the case in behavior analysis. In this respect, Kantor's interbehavioral approach is similar to current frameworks that have been used to analyze family interactions, namely, ecobehavioral (Lutzker, 1984; Rogers-Warren & Warren, 1977) and ecological approaches (Barker, 1963; Bronfenbrenner, 1977). Other frameworks for analysis of multiple variables in family interactions have been the approaches traditionally referred to as "systems interventions." These interventions include strategic (Haley, 1971; Jackson, 1965), functional (Alexander & Barton, 1976), and structural (Minuchin, 1974) family therapies.

Interbehavioral psychology also has been compared with ecological psychology (Rogers-Warren & Fox, 1983). A. K. Rogers-Warren and S. Warren (1977) propose that the ecological approach is more of an emphasis on behavior in its physical and behavioral contexts rather than a unified theory of human behavior. Ecologists such as R. G. Barker (1963) conduct primarily observational research, thus satisfying Kantor's insistence upon the confrontability of subject matter. When one begins with the assumption that all behavior occurs within a context, and this is part of a larger context, ad infinitum, the result is elimination of the artificial boundaries around behavior or phenomena of interest. To this extent, interbehavioral and "ecobehavioral" orientations share the same paradigm for scientific study.

Utility of an Expanded Framework

The inclusion of an interbehavioral or ecological perspective may provide insight in designing effective family interventions. The "family" is a system where intervention into any of its subsystems may affect the larger system in some way. Most intervention programs designed for handicapped children target the mother-child dyad and ignore the larger system of which the dyad is a part (Snell & Beckman-Brinkley, 1984).

There are two logical corollaries that follow from targeting the dyad to the exclusion of the larger system. First, any changes produced in dyadic interaction patterns may affect (positively or negatively) the ecology of the family. If, as is usually the case, the researcher monitors only the dyad, changes taking place at the family level could go undetected. It is important that any negative effects of interventions become immediately apparent so that they can be remediated. We need, therefore, to monitor some portion of the extradyadic system for effects resulting from intervention programs.

Second, there may be extradyadic factors impinging upon the dyad, affecting it in ways we will not be aware of if our focus is solely on the dyad. Some of these extradyadic variables may potentially influence the efficacy of our intervention efforts. If so, conclusions drawn about the results of our intervention may be inaccurate or insufficient until these variables are considered.

One of the principle areas in which the use of an expanded framework might assist intervention efforts is in maintenance and generalization. There is a growing body of literature suggesting that parent-training procedures, once learned, are not always maintained (Baker, Heifetz, & Murphy, 1980; Wahler, 1980). In many families, parents demonstrate competency in behavioral principles and apply them to their child. Follow-up contacts, however, frequently reveal that some parents have stopped using their newly learned skills. Reasons for discontinuation have ranged from family crises, lack of time, and daily interruptions to low rates of positive extrafamilial contacts—all of which are extradyadic variables. This lack of maintenance suggests that interventions at the basic or dyadic level may be sufficient for initial child behavior change but may be insufficient to guarantee continued parent involvement in the face of real or perceived obstacles.

What follows is a review of current behavioral parent-training studies of families with developmentally delayed children. Special note will be taken of the presence or absence of description of extradyadic factors that can potentially mediate intervention efficacy and of the measurement of concurrent effects of training on the family system.

Review of Behavioral Parent-Training Research With Families of Developmentally Delayed Children

Twenty-six current behavioral parent-training studies, reported within the past eleven years, have been analyzed for this review. Following is a critical summary of different research issues including (a) limitations, (b) sample size, (c) subjects, (d) parents, (e) parent trainers, (f) training procedures, (g) data collection, (h) generalization, and (i) maintenance.

Limitations of the Literature

Many of the same problems noted in previous critiques and reviews of behavioral parent-training research (Bijou, 1984; Johnson & Katz, 1973; Lutzker, McGimsey, McRae, & Campbell, 1983) are apparent in studies involving developmentally disabled (DD) children. There is a serious lack of description of both subjects and procedures, making replication and generalizations of treatment results difficult. Although the majority of studies with DD children claimed that some positive change had taken place either in parent or child behavior, omission of direct observational measures made many of these claims difficult to confirm. Another limitation is the apparent neglect by many behavioral parent-training investigators to examine the impact of their intervention on the family system and to examine mediating effects of the family system on the effectiveness of the intervention. It should be pointed out that no single study has all of these faults and that several studies are quite exemplary. As a whole, these studies do offer consistent evidence that behavioral parent-training procedures are effective for many parents of developmentally delayed children.

Sample Size

The twenty-six intervention studies included 1,300 children. Excluding a large follow-up study of 348 children (Schopler, Mesibov, & Baker, 1982), the average number of children per study was 40, the median per study was 30, and the range was 6 to 160 children per study.

Attrition rates are not generally reported in clinical interventions studies. Such data are important and should be presented because it is possible that those families who drop out of treatment might have been the least successful had they continued in treatment; they would have decreased the overall success rate of the program. Of those studies that reported an attrition rate, the average rate was about 15 percent.

Subjects

The children represented in these various studies had a variety of handicapping conditions. Classifications included mental retardation, developmental disabilities, autism, and often severe language disabilities. The children's IQ ranged from normal to profoundly mentally retarded. The majority of the subjects were within the mild to severe range of mental retardation. Several studies neglected to include information on the child's intellectual functioning, and only a very few presented information about the child's adaptive behavior level.

Subjects' ages ranged from as young as three weeks up to twenty-six years of age, with most being in the two- to fourteen-year range. The average age was approximately 6.5 years. Child gender was mentioned infrequently, but in those studies in which it was reported, 78 percent were male and 22 percent were female. This difference may be determined largely by the observation that developmental disabilities are more common in males than in females (Reed & Anderson, 1973).

A surprising pattern in the majority of studies was the inattention to descriptions of inappropriate behavior although the goal was to reduce inappropriate behavior and remediate behavioral deficits. Only a few studies included even a brief description of the subject's inappropriate behavior. Descriptions including "topography" and "function" would appear to be important in any intervention since it influences the amount of programming that a parent would need to learn.

Parents

Since parents normally are the direct focus of behavioral parent training, it seems somewhat dismaying that so few demographic data are presented on them, especially because demographics can relate to behavioral parent-training outcome (Griest & Forehand, 1982; Wahler, 1980). Nonetheless, of those studies that indicated parental gender, 95 percent of the parents were female and 5 percent male.

Socioeconomic status (SES) also was reported infrequently; when it was presented it appears that most parents were middle class. Parental age ranged from sixteen to fifty-four years, with the average being 37.5 years. Most parents had completed high school, with an average of 13.5 years of education. Only one study (Baker, Prieto-Bayard, & McCurry, 1984) specifically targeted low SES families, where parents had on the average finished fifth grade. In the few studies that mentioned marital status, 85 percent of the parents were reported as being married. Ethnic group membership and cultural factors were reported too infrequently to determine the proportion of parents from any particular group. In conclusion, it appears that most parents have completed high school, are married, and are in their mid- to late thirties.

Parent Trainers

Parent trainers were also described poorly in the majority of the studies (cf. Lutzker, McGimsey, McRae, & Campbell, 1983). Trainer's age, ethnic group membership, and gender were infrequently mentioned. These are variables that might have an effect on the degree of rapport attained between parent and therapist. Of those trainers described, all had bachelor's degrees, and the majority were graduate students or doctoral-level psychologists. Most were reported to have had extensive experience in working with handicapped children or their families. Overall, there was a general lack of information about the agents who actually provided training to the parents.

Training Procedures

Many of the twenty-six studies contained descriptions of training procedures that were so marginal as to make replication of the study difficult, if not impossible. Attempts to measure the application of parent-training procedures were likewise infrequent. Only two studies (Koegel, Schreibman, Britten, Burke, & O'Neill, 1982; Lovaas, Koegel, Simmons, & Long, 1973) reported monitoring parent behavior to ascertain that parents were actually learning and implementing parenting skills. Two other studies were also criterion-referenced (McClannahan, Krantz, & McGee, 1982; Revill & Blunden, 1979), but they used child rather than parent behavior as the gauge to determine whether parents had actually learned new skills. The assumption in this case appears to be that if child behavior is changing, then parent behavior must also be changing. Though it is important to use actual data to gauge program success, a more direct measure of the independent variable (parent behavior) would be to observe the parents' behavior. In two-thirds of the studies there was a prescribed number of training sessions for the parents, regardless of parent or child progress. The number of sessions in these studies ranged from six to sixteen, with the average number of sessions at approximately ten.

Parent-training program components were described in about half of the studies; these included parent-training manuals and programmed materials, lecture format, group discussions, feedback, modeling, individual trainer time with parents, role-playing, and direct coaching. "Booster shots"—when the trainer assists parents after formal training has ended —was mentioned in only two studies. These same studies were the only two to use a criterion for the parents to progress through the program (Koegel, et al., 1982; Lovaas et al., 1973).

Control groups or controlled baseline designs were included in approximately half the studies. Outcomes of these studies indicated that behavioral parent training was superior to no treatment. Comparison of behavioral parent training to other forms of treatment was done in the study by Tavormina (1975), and found it superior to reflective or thematic group counseling.

Six studies included a component analysis. B. Baker and colleagues (1980), D. Clark and colleagues (1982), and L. Heifetz (1977) evaluated the use of instructional manuals as well as the effects of differing amounts of professional assistance to parents. They found that the use of manuals alone was as effective as using manuals *plus* group training *plus* individual home visits for the mothers, even though it inspired less confidence. R. Brightman, B. Baker, D. Clark, and S. Ambrose (1982) found group and individual parent-training formats equally effective. A. Hudson (1982) compared the results of a specific behavior focus group, a specific focus plus the use of modeling group, and a group that utilized both of the above procedures plus role-playing. Hudson concluded that principles of social learning theory did not improve parent performance and that modeling and role-playing were not necessary components for effective parent performances. S. O'Dell, J. Flynn, and L. Benlolo (1977) also found that teaching parents learning principles did not appear to increase parent performance.

Data Collection

Data-collection procedures varied from study to study, and all but a few studies employed multiple outcome measures. Types of measurement procedures included direct observation of child and parent behavior, objective psychological measures such as parent or child IQ scores, and parent self-report measures. Few of the studies included direct observational measures of behavior. Instead, assessment covered parent skill (collected through the observation of independent observers); child behavior change (collected by either the parent or directly observed by an independent observer); clinical measures, such as IQ or developmental scores for the child and personality profiles for the parents; and information volunteered by parents in the form of questionnaires, interviews, and a checklist of parent and/or child behavior.

Obstacles to training were assessed in several studies—by interview in one (Holmes, Hemsley, Rickett, & Likierman, 1982) and by use of an "Obstacles to Training Scale" in two others (Baker et al., 1980; Clark et al., 1982). Commonly reported obstacles included lack of time, child's behavior problems, parental perceived inability and need for support, and parental dislike of the behavioral philosophy.

Side effects of training were discussed in several of the studies. For example, Holmes and colleagues (1982) found that parents reported they were better able to cope with their child and that they could use the parent trainer as someone to talk to about family difficulties, and Koegel and colleagues (1982) found that parent training increased the family's leisure time from 40 minutes per day to 140 minutes per day.

Generalization

Generalization is obviously an important facet of any intervention program. Stokes and Baer (1977) define generalization as "the occurrence of relevant behavior under different, nontraining conditions (i.e., across subjects, settings, people, behaviors, or time)" (p. 350). In parent training there are two types of generalization to be assessed: that of the child (for example, the generalization of child behaviors trained by the parent) and that of the parent (such as the generalization of parent behaviors produced by the parent-training procedures).

In the few studies that assessed generalization of child behavior, there was little evidence that it had occurred. Generalization of parent behavior was generally programmed by either "mediating generalization" (training general principles), by providing "sufficient examplars" (providing multiple examples of specific behaviors), or both.

Types of parent generalization included setting generality (the transfer of training from one setting to another), behavior generality (the parent's independent teaching of multiple behaviors to the child), and parent generality (the generalization of learned behaviors from one parent to another). Types of measures of these three categories of generalization included direct observation, parent self-report, and tests prompting responses to hypothetical situations involving the child. Overall, the same results with generalization occurred in these studies as in the rest of the intervention literature—positive in some instances, negative in others.

Maintenance

Maintenance, the durability of initial behavior change over time, is another extremely important phenomenon to assess in any intervention program. The fact that parents are in daily contact with these children and can implement behavioral contingencies increases the likelihood of learned skills being retained. However, the assumption to which this leads is a problem. The assumption is that once parents have successfully learned how to modify their child's behavior, positive behaviors of the child will automatically motivate and maintain the parents' newly acquired skills. Let us consider this assumption in light of the twenty-six studies reviewed.

Of the twenty-six studies, one-half included some follow-up measure. The range of time covered between cessation of formal training procedures and follow-up ranged from one month to twelve years, although most were in the one- to fourteen-month follow-up range. The median amount of time reported for follow-up was six months. Parents were the main informants for follow-up data, usually through self-report measures such as questionnaires or interviews. In most of the studies a continuation of treatment results for the child was reported, but most parents recounted that they had switched from using formal training procedures to using some type of incidental training procedures. It is important in considering the report of maintenance to know that the data were usually reported by parents and that investigators rarely arranged for independent evaluation of the child behavior.

Summary

This review of twenty-six behavioral parent-training studies for families of developmentally delayed children affirms the same difficulties noted in reviews that have focused on behavioral parent training of nonhandicapped children (e.g., Johnson & Katz, 1973). These difficulties include a lack of description of subjects and of training procedures, a lack of measurement of the independent variable, a focus on dyadic versus systems interaction patterns, and difficulties with generalization and maintenance. However, taken as an aggregate, evidence is presented that makes a strong case for initial acquisition of parenting skills, a moderate case for increased family functioning, and a moderate case for maintenance of child behavior gains as a result of behavioral parent training.

Aside from prompting authors to include better descriptions of their subjects and training procedures, several major weaknesses remain to be discussed. First is the need for investigators to measure both child and parent behavior to determine the relationship between these two variables rather than making nondata-based assumptions about causality. A second weakness is the lack of consistency in utilizing direct measurement of child and parent behavior as a standard outcome measure. A third weakness is the usual emphasis on dyadic interactions rather than on the system of which the dyad is but a part.

Most of the studies reviewed included some description of variables deemed important in a well-designed behavioral parent study, but overall, few studies included even a majority of these variables. Recalling the evidence that parent-training outcome is influenced by variables such as those described above, and recalling the lack of generalization and moderate success in maintenance, it behooves the investigator to begin to take into account these previously neglected phenomena.

Once again, it is averred that an expanded theoretical framework such as that offered by Kantor (1959) might assist the investigator in producing a more effective, durable intervention that is harmonious with the family ecology. Several parent-training investigators have produced research that comes out of an expanded framework, and some actually used Kantor's writings as a working model. The following section includes a brief description of some of the more innovative research produced by these parent-training investigators.

Parent-Training Investigators Utilizing an Expanded Framework

Several parent-training interventionists take into account more than the usual analysis of mother-child interactions. Although not all of these investigators work with families of handicapped children, results of their research apply to these families because of the complex demands placed on the parents.

R. G. Wahler and his colleagues (e.g., Wahler, 1980; Wahler & Afton, 1980; Wahler, Leske, & Rogers, 1979) are perhaps best known for their work with insular mothers. While working with low-income mothers of socially aggressive and oppositional children, Wahler and his colleagues found that these mothers were able to induce change in their child's behavior initially, but there was limited generalization and maintenance of parent-training efforts. An analysis of their limited success revealed that extrafamilial factors were influencing training outcome results. Through the use of a checklist that assessed daily social contacts, Wahler and his colleagues found that on days when the mother had high rates of positive extrafamilial contacts, her interactions with her child were contingent and appropriate. However, on days when the preceding twenty-four-hour period was characterized by low rates of postive extrafamilial contacts and by high rates of negative contacts with extended family members and social helping agencies, the mother's interactions with her child were predominantly negative. Wahler has utilized the setting-event concept to explain the effects of parent insularity on parent-child interaction patterns. This research is clearly relevant to families of handicapped children, because these parents are also often characterized by insularity effects (McAllister, Butler, & Lei, 1973).

J. Breiner and D. L. Young (in press) adopted Wahler's insularity measures and compared mothers of nonhandicapped, noncompliant children with mothers of developmentally delayed, noncompliant children. Their results indicated that there was a lower rate of social interaction in the mothers of the delayed children. This research using insularity measures extends the setting-event concept to research involving handicapped children and provides additional empirical support for the notion of social isolation in parents of handicapped children.

G. R. Patterson and his colleagues have also worked with socially aggressive and oppositional children and their families. Patterson has focused on the spiraling patterns of aversive interactions between parent and child, which he called "coercive cycles." These cycles generally exist in families in which the father has a limited role, the mother has relatively little skill in child management, and there are high rates of mother-child contact. These factors may function as setting events for coercive interactions between mother and child. Patterson has also examined the role of depression, parental mood, and personality characteristics on parenting ability. In addition, intervention efforts from this research group are extended toward the entire family network rather than exclusively to the mother-child dyad.

J. R. Lutzker and his colleagues (Lutzker, 1984; Tertinger, Greene, & Lutzker, in press) describe research that is modeled after an ecobehavioral approach (Rogers-Warren & Warren, 1977). Their work with abusive and neglectful families included analyses of the physical environment and its relationship to child abuse. Lutzker's research group has also provided multilevel intervention programs for their families. These programs include not only a standard behavioral parent-training component but also occupational and marital counseling, as well as additional interventions deemed appropriate for each particular family.

The research of Griest & Forehand (1982) and Griest, Wells, & Forehand (1979) has focused on young noncompliant children and their mothers. This research group has produced ample evidence that parent-training results can be mediated by parental characteristics such as depression and parental adjustment. They have also reported the effects of an intervention that they have termed parent enhancement therapy. This particular intervention consists of teaching the standard parent-training techniques plus teaching the parent to deal with child expectations, parental mood, partner communication, problem solving, and relationships with nonfamily members. Results indicated that this intervention produced better treatment effects and better maintenance than behavioral parent training alone.

R. L. Koegel and his colleagues (Koegel et al., 1982; Lovaas et al., 1973) have worked with autistic children and their families. This research group has made use of assessment devices that target the effect of their intervention on family and parental functioning. Family functioning has been assessed by scores on the MMPI, the Dyadic Adjustment Scale (a marital adjustment scale), the Family Environment Scale, and by use of a daily activity diary detailing the manner in which the parents spent their day. The most striking results obtained were that after parent training, parent leisure time increased from 40 to 140 minutes per day, a substantial increase.

Summary

The intent of this chapter has been to review parent-training research on families with handicapped children in view of the need to expand the behavioral framework to a systems perspective. As Kantor (1959) proposed, a systems viewpoint enlarges the unit or field of analysis beyond the basic three-term contingency to include many impinging variables in the family context. A shortcoming of most current parent-training programs is the exclusion of surrounding social variables. The research, in affirming Kantor's model, demonstrates that training outcome relates to extradyadic factors such as parental characteristics, family crises, economic status, and low rates of positive extrafamilial social contacts. There have been, however, few investigators who have taken these variables into account when designing their interventions.

The fact the parent-training outcome has proven to be influenced by extradyadic variables is even more ostensible in families with handicapped children. These families often experience greater stress than families with nonhandicapped children. Partly because there is a large number of factors impinging upon these families, and partly because these factors have been shown to influence training results, it seems especially important to take these factors into consideration when designing and evaluating an intervention program.

Several parent-training investigators have examined more than the usual dyadic interactions by considering extradyadic factors. There appears, then, a growing trend in the literature toward more system-oriented research investigations. One might hope this trend will lead to a comprehensive framework that combines the broader approach of Kantor with that based on the three-term contingency.

References

Adesso, V. , and J. Lipson. 1981. Group training of parents as therapists for their children. *Behavior Therapy* 12: 625–33.

Alexander, J., and C. Barton. 1976. Behavioral systems therapy for families. In D. H. Olson (Ed.), *Treating relationships*. Lake Mills, Iowa: Graphic.

Baker, B. 1976. Parent involvement in programming for developmentally disabled children. In L. Lloyd (Ed.), *Communication assessment and intervention strategies*. Baltimore: University Park Press.

Baker, B. 1980. Training parents as teachers of their developmentally delayed children. In S. Salzinger, J. Antrobus, & J. Glick (Eds.), *The ecosystem of the sick child.* New York: Academic Press.

Baker, B., A. J. Brightman, L. J. Heifetz, and D. Murphy. 1976. *Steps to independence series: Behavior problems, early self-help skills, intermediate self-help skills, advanced self-help skills, toilet training.* Champaign, Ill. Research Press.

Baker, B., L. Heifetz, and D. Murphy. 1980. Behavioral training for parents of mentally retarded children: One-year follow-up. *American Journal of Mental Deficiency* 85: 31–38.

Baker, B., M. Prieto-Bayard, and M. McCurry. 1984. Lower socioeconomic status families and programs for training parents of retarded children. In J. M. Berg (Ed.), *Perspectives and progress in mental retardation.* Baltimore: University Park Press.

Bandura, A. 1969. *Principles of behavior modification.* New York: Holt, Rinehart & Winston.

Barker, R. G. 1963. *The stream of behavior.* New York: Appleton-Century-Crofts.

Barnard, J., E. Christopherson, and M. Wolf. 1977. Teaching children appropriate shopping behavior through parent training in the supermarket. *Journal of Applied Behavior Analysis* 10: 49–59.

Baum, C., and R. Forehand. 1981. Long term follow-up assessment of parent training by use of multiple outcome measures. *Behavior Therapy* 12: 643–52.

Bergreen, S. 1971. A study of the mental health of near relatives of twenty multihandicapped children. *Acta Paed Scandinavia* 2: 16–23.

Berkowitz, B., and A. Graziano. 1972. Training parents as behavior therapists: A reveiw. *Behaviour Research and* Therapy 10: 297–317.

Bijou, S. W. 1984. Parent training: Actualizing the critical conditions of early childhood development. In R. Dangel and R. Polster (Eds.), *Parent training: Foundations of research and practice.* New York: Guilford Press.

Bijou, S. W., and D. M. Baer. 1961. *Child development: A systematic and empirical theory.* New York: Appleton.

Breiner, J., and D. L. Young. In press. Social interaction: A comparison of mothers with noncompliant, nondelayed and developmentally delayed children. *Child and Family Behavior Therapy.*

Brightman, R., B. Baker, D. Clark, and S. Ambrose. 1982. Effectiveness of alternative parent training formats. *Journal of Behavior Therapy and Experimental Psychiatry* 13: 113–17.

Bronfenbrenner, U. 1977. Toward an experimental ecology of human behavior. *American Psychologist* 32: 513–31.

Brown, W. H., W. Bryson-Brockmann, and J. J. Fox. 1984, November. *Differentiating setting events from discriminative stimuli: An interbehavioral perspective.* Paper presented at the first annual meeting of the South Eastern Association for Behavior Analysis, Myrtle Beach, South Carolina.

Burden, R. L. 1980. Measuring the effects of stress on the mothers of handicapped infants: Must depression always follow? *Child: Health Care and Development* 6: 111–25.

Butler, J. 1976. The toilet training success of parents after reading *Toilet Training in Less Than a Day. Behavior Therapy* 7: 185–91.

Clark, D., B. Baker, and L. Heifetz. 1982. Behavioral training for parents of mentally retarded children: Prediction of outcome. *American Journal of Mental Deficiency* 87: 14–19.

Cummings, S., H. Bayley, and H. Rie. 1966. Effects of the child's deficiency on the mother: A study of mothers of mentally retarded, chronically ill, and neurotic children. *American Journal of Orthopsychiatry* 36: 595–608.

Daurelle, L. A. and J. J. Fox. 1984, November. *An interbehavioral perspective on parent training of developmentally delayed children*. Paper presented at the first annual meeting of the South Eastern Association for Behavior Analysis, Myrtle Beach, South Carolina.

Davis, F. 1967. Family process in mental retardation. *American Journal of Psychiatry* 124: 96–106.

DeMyer, M., and P. Goldberg. 1983. Family needs of the autistic adolescent. In E. Schopler and G. B. Mesibov (Eds.), *Autism in adolescents and adults*. New York: Plenum.

Farber, B. 1959. Effects of a severely retarded child on family integration. *Monographs of the Society for Research in Child Development* 24: Serial No. 71.

Farber, B. 1968. *Mental retardation: Its social context and social consequences*. Boston: Houghton Mifflin.

Farber, B., and D. B. Ryckman. 1965. Effects of severely mentally retarded children on family relationships. *Mental Retardation Abstracts* 2: 1–17.

Forehand, R., E. Sturgis, R. McMahon, D. Aguar, K. Green, K. Wells, and J. Breiner. 1979. Parent behavioral training to modify child noncompliance: Treatment generalization across time and from home to school. *Behavior Modification* 3: 3–25.

Fowle, C. M. 1968. The effect of the severely mentally retarded child on his family. *American Journal of Mental Deficiency* 73: 468–73.

Friedrich, W. N., and W. L. Friedrich. 1981. Psychosocial assets of parents of handicapped and nonhandicapped children. *American Journal of Mental Deficiency* 85: 551–53.

Glogower, F., and E. Sloop. 1976. Two strategies of group training of parents as effective behavior modifiers. *Behavior Therapy* 7: 177–84.

Griest, D., and R. Forehand. 1982. How can I get any parent training done with all these other problems going on?: The role of family variables in child behavior therapy. *Child and Family Behavior Therapy* 4: 73–80.

Griest, D. L., R. Forehand, T. Rogers, J. Breiner, W. Furey, and C. A. Williams. 1982. Effects of parent enhancement therapy on the treatment outcome and generalization of a parent training program. *Behaviour Research and Therapy* 20: 429–36.

Greist, D., K. Wells, and R. Forehand. 1979. An examination of predictors of maternal perception of maladjustment in clinic-referred children. *Journal of Abnormal Psychology* 88: 277–81.

Grossman, F. K. 1972. *Brothers and sisters of retarded children*. Syracuse: Syracuse University Press.

Guthrie, E. 1935. *The psychology of learning*. New York: Harper.

Haley, J. 1971. Family therapy: A radical change. In J. Haley (Ed.), *Changing families*. New York: Grune & Stratton.

Hawkins, R., R. Peterson, E. Schweid, and S. Bijou. 1966. Behavior therapy in the home: Amelioration of problem parent-child relations with the parent in a therapeutic role. *Journal of Experimental Child Psychology* 4: 99–107.

Heifetz, L. 1977. Behavioral training for parents of retarded children: Alternative formats based on instructional manuals. *American Journal of Mental Deficiency* 82: 194–203.

Holmes, N., R. Hemsley, L. Rickett, and H. Likierman. 1982. Parents as co-therapists: Their perceptions of a home-based behavioral treatment for autistic children. *Journal of Autism and Developmental Disorders* 12: 331–42.

Hudson, A. 1982. Training parents of developmentally handicapped children: A component analysis. *Behavior Therapy* 13: 325–33.

Jackson, D. D. 1965. The study of the family. *Family Process* 4: 1–20.

Jeffries, R. 1983. *Impact of the handicapped child on the family.* Unpublished manuscript, George Peabody College of Vanderbilt University.

Johnson, C., and R. Katz. 1973. Using parents as change agents for their children: A review. *Journal of Child Psychology and Psychiatry* 14: 181–200.

Johnson, S., and G. Lobitz. 1974. Parental manipulations of child behavior in home observations. *Journal of Applied Behavior Analysis* 7: 23–31.

Kantor, J. R. 1959. *Interbehavioral psychology*, rev. ed. Granville, Ohio: Principia Press.

Kantor, J. R. 1966. Feelings and emotions as scientific events. *Psychological Record* 16: 377–404.

Koegel, R. L., L. Schreibman, K. Britten, J. C. Burke, and R. E. O'Neill. 1982. A comparison of parent training to direct child treatment. In R. L. Koegel, A. Rincover, and A. L. Egel (Eds.), *Educating and understanding autistic children.* Houston: College-Hill Press.

Leigland, S. 1984. On "setting events" and related concepts. *The Behavior Analyst* 7: 41–45.

Lovaas, O. I., R. Koegel, J. Simmons, and J. Long. 1973. Some generalizations and follow-up measures on autistic children in behavior therapy. *Journal of Applied Behavior Analysis,* 6:131–66.

Lutzker, J. R. 1984. Project 12-Ways: Treating child abuse and neglect from an eco-behavioral perspective. In R. F. Dangel and R. A. Polster (Eds.), *Parent training: Foundations of research and practice.* New York: Guilford Press.

Lutzker, J. R., J. McGimsey, S. McRae, and R. Campbell. 1983. Behavioral parent training: There's so much more to do. *The Behavior Therapist* 6: 110–12.

McAllister, R. J., E. W. Butler and T. J. Lei. 1973. Patterns of social interaction among families of behaviorally retarded children. *Journal of Marriage and the Family* 35: 93–100.

McClannahan, L., P. Krantz, and G. McGee. 1982. Parents as therapists for autistic children: A model for effective parent training. *Analysis and Intervention in Developmental Disabilities* 2:223–52.

Michael, J. L. 1982. Distinguishing between discriminative and motivational functions of stimuli. *Journal of the Experimental Analysis of Behavior* 37: 149–55.

Minuchin, S. 1974. *Families and family therapy.* Cambridge, Mass.: Harvard University Press.

Mira, M. 1970. Results of a behavior modification training program for parents and teachers. *Behaviour Research and Therapy,* 8: 308–11.

O'Dell, S. 1974. Training parents in behavior modification: A review. *Psychological Bulletin* 81: 418–33.

O'Dell, S., J. Flynn, and L. Benlolo. 1977. A comparison of parent training techniques in child behavior modification. *Journal of Behavior Therapy and Experimental Psychiatry* 8: 261–68.

Oltmanns, T., J. Broderick, and K. D. O'Leary. 1977. Marital adjustment and the efficacy of behavior therapy with children. *Journal of Consulting and Clinical Psychology* 45: 724–29.

Patterson, G. R. 1971. Behavioral intervention procedures in the classroom and in the home. In A. E. Bergin and S. L. Garfield (Eds.), *Handbook of psychotherapy and behavior change*. New York: Wiley.

Patterson, G. R., and M. E. Gullion. 1976. *Living with children: New methods for parents and teachers*, rev. ed. Champaign, Ill.: Research Press.

Poznanski, E. 1969. Psychiatric difficulties in siblings of handicapped children. *Pediatrics* 8: 232–34.

Reed, S. C. and V. A. Anderson. 1973. Effects of changing sexuality on the gene pool. In F. F. de la Cruz and G. D. LeVeck (Eds.), *Human sexuality and the mentally retarded*. New York: Brunner/Mazel.

Reisinger, J., G. Frangia, and E. Hoffman. 1976. Toddler management training: Generalization and marital status. *Journal of Behavior Therapy and Experimental Psychiatry* 7: 335–40.

Revill, S., and R. Blunden. 1979. A home training service for pre-school developmentally handicapped. *Behaviour Research and Therapy* 17: 207–14.

Risley, T. R. 1968. The effects and side effects of punishing the autistic behaviors of a deviant child. *Journal of Applied Behavior Analysis* 1: 21–34.

Rogers-Warren, A. K., and J. J. Fox. 1983, September. *Behavioral parent training research: Contributions to an ecological analysis of families with handicapped children*. Paper presented at the NICHD conference on "Research on Families with Retarded Persons," Raleigh, North Carolina.

Rogers-Warren, A. K. and S. Warren. (Eds.). 1977. *Ecological perspectives in behavior analysis*. Baltimore: University Park Press.

Rose, S. 1974a. Group training of parents as behavior modifiers. *Social Work* 19: 156–62.

Rose, S. 1974b. Training parents in groups as behavior modifiers of their mentally retarded children. *Journal of Behavior Therapy and Experimental Psychiatry* 5: 135–40.

Russo, S. 1964. Adaptations in behavioral therapy with children. *Behaviour Research and Therapy* 2: 43–47.

Schopler, E., G. Mesibov, and A. Baker. 1982. Evaluation of treatment for autistic children and their parents. *Journal of the American Academy of Child Psychiatry* 21: 262–67.

Skinner, B. F. 1953. *Science and human behavior*. London: Macmillan.

Skinner, B. F. 1974. *About behaviorism*. New York: Alfred A. Knopf.

Sloane, H. N., M. Johnston, and S. Bijou. 1967. Successive modification of aggressive behavior and aggressive fantasy play by management of contingencies. *Journal of Child Psychology and Psychiatry* 8: 217–26.

Snell, M. E., and S. Beckman-Brinkley. 1984. Family involvement in intervention with children having severe handicaps. *Journal of the Association for the Severely Handicapped* 9: 213–30.

Stokes, T. F., and D. M. Baer. 1977. An implicit technology of generalization. *Journal of Applied Behavior Analysis* 10: 349–67.

Straughan, H. 1964. Treatment with mother and child in the playroom. *Behaviour Research and Therapy* 2: 37–41.

Tavormina, J. 1975. Relative effectiveness of behavioral and reflective group counseling with parents of mentally retarded children. *Journal of Consulting and Clinical Psychology* 43: 22–31.

Tavormina, J., T. J. Boll, N. J. Dunn, R. L. Luscomb, and J. R. Taylor. 1981. Psychosocial effects on parents of raising a physically handicapped child. *Journal of Abnormal Child Psychology* 9: 121–31.

Tertinger, D., B. Greene, and J. R. Lutzker. In press. Home safety: Development and validation of one component of an ecobehavioral treatment program for abused and neglected children. *Journal of Applied Behavior Analysis.*

Tew, B. J., K. M. Laurence, H. Payne, and K. Rawnsley. 1977. Marital stability following the birth of a child with spina bifida. *British Journal of Psychiatry* 131: 79–82.

Tharp, R., and R. Wetzel. 1969. *Behavior modification in the natural environment.* New York: Academic Press.

Wahler, R. G. 1980. The insular mother: Her problems in parent-child treatment. *Journal of Applied Behavior Analysis* 13: 207–19.

Wahler, R. G., and A. D. Afton. 1980. Attentional processes in insular and noninsular mothers. *Child Behavior Therapy* 2: 25–41.

Wahler, R. G., and J. J. Fox. 1981. Setting events in applied behavior analysis: Toward a conceptual and methodological expansion. *Journal of Applied Behavior Analysis* 14: 327–38.

Wahler, R. G., and M. G. Graves. 1983. Setting events in social networks: Ally or enemy in child behavior therapy? *Behavior Therapy* 14: 19–36.

Wahler, R. G. and D. M. Hann. In press. A behavioral systems perspective on childhood psychopathology: Expanding the three term operant contingency. In N. Krasnegor (Ed.), *Child health care behavior.*

Wahler, R. G., G. Leske, and E. Rogers. 1979. The insular family: A deviance support system for oppositional children. In L. A. Hamerlynck (Ed.), *Behavioral systems for the developmentally disabled. 1. School and family environments.* New York: Brunner/Mazel.

Williams, C. 1959. The elimination of tantrum behavior by extinction procedures. *Journal of Abnormal and Social Psychology* 59: 269.

12

Community-Based Psychological Services for Developmentally Retarded Persons

Mary Ann Scafasci

Historically, the behavioral systems approach has encountered the more traditional methods of referral service delivery at the theoretical and technological
levels. Referral systems generally consist of interrelations between human service
agencies within a community by way of formal or informal contract. Networking
models that address the need for interagency referral consider this system a
departure from the orthodox practice of service exclusion (Janicki, Castellani,
& Norris, 1983). Advances in networking seemingly expand opportunities for
interdisciplinary participation in a client's overall program, but in reality this
amounts to a glorified subway transporting clients from one terminal to another
without communication between stops. The alternative networking model presented in this chapter derives from the systems psychology of J. R. Kantor
(1924). This approach stresses not only mechanisms of referral process but, more
important, the essential role of "field events" (concurrent changes) in the client's
life. The behavioral systems approach especially provides direction in coordinating services for developmentally retarded persons residing in the community.

This chapter first overviews historical antecedents to the interbehavioral systems approach to community-based services. Second, contrast is shown between
traditional methodology and the interbehavioral perspective. Next, the psychologist as part of the interbehavioral field is examined, including critical issues in
clinical application. Finally, in tying the pieces together, a case study demonstrates some key considerations of interbehavioral interventions with developmentally retarded persons.

Historical Perspective

It is helpful to trace the history of psychological services because it mirrors
the historical evolution of general trends in psychological service delivery. As

in any system, the progression is not clear-cut or totally innovative in that emphasis for treatment and habilitation of retarded individuals has evolved from several modalities along a continuum of theoretical progression. Methods for treatment have varied and overlapped, not just during "early" years of research with this population but more recently as well. Early emphasis was upon basic models of custodial, institutional care. Several accounts already exist on pre-humanitarian treatment of retarded persons and their overall image in society (Kazdin, 1978; Szasz, 1961). Retarded persons were viewed as a population having a condition that was neither treatable nor curable. Although this was the general rule, exceptions such as the the the single-case study of the "Wild Boy of Aveyron" (Whitman & Scibak, 1981) questioned the educability of a child despite his gross deficits in socially appropriate behavior; questions also arose concerning environmental causes.

The formal introduction of behavior modification or operant psychology (Whitman & Scibak, 1981) provided a means to bridge a service delivery gap with this population. Previously, obvious difficulties were found with implementation of traditional forms of therapy such as "catharsis," "insight," and "self-actualization" (Matson, 1984; Nuffield, 1983). Greater problems were evident for untreated individuals who were nonverbal or who were classified in severe to profound ranges of retardation (Matson, 1984). Largely because of treatment failures and dehumanization, behavior modification filled a clinical gap through its demonstrated experimental viability.

As late as the 1960s, the focus in institutional settings with regard to treatment for this population changed to this "new technology" of behavior modification. The experimental effectiveness of behavioral procedures across a wide variety of populations and problems was now being brought into the institution for further evaluation and research. Emphasis was upon demonstrating the educability of retarded individuals through teaching appropriate and independent self-care skills (such as toileting, bathing), as well as the elimination of socially defined inappropriate behaviors (e.g., self-abuse, physical aggression toward others). The sophistication of this technology thus evolved from "simplistic" applications of basic reinforcement principles and eliminative procedures to more complex methodologies such as differential reinforcement of alternative behavior (DRA) and differential reinforcement of zero-based behavior (DRO).

T. L. Whitman and J. W. Scibak (1981) detailed the prevalence of published studies on behavior modification with the developmentally retarded population. The profound increase of technology since the early 1960s focuses upon a wide variety of target behaviors, change procedures, and deficit levels of subjects (classified as mild to profound). While the premise of applied behavioral technology has been built upon experimental laboratory research, not all studies within the traditional behavioral framework have managed to provide systematic evidence of the applicability of techniques across settings and of techniques that produce long-term effects (Whitman & Scibak, 1981).

One important consequence of widespread acceptance of behavior modification was the change in the definition of developmentally retarded persons. This change was reflected in the orientation of care and service provided to this population. Developmentally retarded persons became "educable" and the focus of treatment evolved from institutionalized custodial care to normalized habilitation in the community setting. Emphasis shifted from defining the developmentally disturbed as organically or "constitutionally" deficient, and therefore untreatable, to recognition of behavioral and developmental deficits that would allow potential for education and treatment.

Eventually, even the terminology began to reflect changes in theory of treatment for this population. Initially, emphasis was upon *mental* retardation. The basic premise for early theories was rooted in "mentalistic" beliefs, including such concepts as native intelligence, personality, organic dysfunction, traits, genetics, and heredity. And despite their tenuous constructional status, these constructs became prime descriptors of actual conditions. This led to the treatment of retardation as an indicator of some hypothetical internal deficiency either biological (e.g., the brain) or mental (e.g., intelligence or learning ability).

Following this orientation, a means to ascertain or measure mental deficiency continued to develop. Consequently, there was a rise and prolific use of normatively based intelligence tests with this population. Efforts to quantify defective abilities added to the reification of these hypothetical mental structures. Such attempts to measure levels of "intellectual" impairment were (and still are) utilized to quantify and define "mental deficiency."

Concurrent with these trends, research and the use of chemical treatments of purported mental conditions were also advancing. Nonbehaviorally based theories of retardation had continued to focus upon traditional medical model interventions. The use of medications to "control" behavior and other physiological prosthetics were the prescription to compensate for inner or intrinsic deficits seen as comprising permanent handicaps.

The behavioral movement considerably altered the face of treatment for the developmentally disabled, and it sometimes resulted in more blemishes than had appeared before. However, methods of behavior modification developed into a relatively simple practice and thoroughly advanced the humanistic image of the disabled. Important contributions in the behavioral movement got away from traditional therapist-patient models of interaction. S. Minuchin (1974) observed that the environmental and social context of the individual was incorporated into any therapeutic process. This created a need for the involvement of family in therapy and a redefinition of the "site of pathology." The therapist's observation of group and social interactions sought dynamics within natural contexts, as opposed to simply describing these interactions. Consequently, the potential targets for therapeutic intervention shifted from the individual to the family as a unit (or its individual members), as well as to other social agencies (such as schools) which participated and contributed to the individual's "field" of activity (Minuchin, 1974; Patterson, 1975).

Similarly, G. R. Patterson (1975) contributed to the changing model of service delivery through his advocacy of the psychologist as a consultant to provide training to "nonprofessionals" (e.g., families, teachers). This is largely an attempt to address problem behaviors and skill deficits within their natural settings. Not only does Patterson recognize the need to train behavior modifiers (change agents), but he considers this training a function of ongoing interactions between trainer and disabled resident. In other words, the first step is predominantly to change the behavior of the change agent in order to impact upon the behavior of the client.

The Interbehavioral Perspective

The shortcomings of traditional treatment models for this population call for alternative models integrating all functional aspects of the intervention. This is why an integrated field theory can contribute to the developmental disabilities areas. Individually, interbehavioral constructs are not new or revolutionary. However, it is the integration and systematization of this model that strengthen clinical applicability. G. Berkson summarizes the model as "descriptions of the environment as well as the behavior of individuals in them (and their consequent interactions) [which] constitute the phenomena to be studied . . . and direct us toward the use of multivariate and interactional methods of design" (1978, p. 406).

An interbehavioral or systems approach extends beyond applications of basic principles to include the utilization of *varied and comprehensive* data-collection mechanisms to record and identify multiple response patterns. "Field behaviorism . . . approaches psychological studies from the standpoint of confrontable events in the same way as any natural science does. The field behaviorist becomes interested in the interbehavior of organisms under defininte environing conditions and proceeds to investigate them in a manner suitable to the original events and in conformity with the technological means available" (Kantor, 1968, p. 161).

This may be best illustrated in reviewing the use of response decrement procedures such as punishment and extinction. Typically, such techniques are understood as reducing a single response under investigation; however, the interbehavioral perspective emphasizes that single-response descriptions are incomplete. Instead, interacting responses are components of interbehavioral fields:

The main assumption of the analysis of response decrements in terms of interacting behavioral patterns is that a decrement in a measured response implicates at least one other response. The interaction response patterns view emphasizes that decremental effects require increments in alternative or antagonistic responses . . . In contrast to single-response analysis, the point of departure for the present approach is multiple-response methodology that reveals various and complex local response interaction patterns that are not amenable to description in terms of one or two underlying states or properties . . . The theoretical foundation for multibehavioral methodology is field behaviorism, and the methodological basis is descriptive functional analysis." (Delprato, 1983 p. 4)

Following this formulation, we dispose of the need to work under the restrictions of a simple cause-effect/stimulus-response model. Kantor made the same observation:

The alternative to the causal construction is the interbehavioral field. An event is regarded as a field of factors all of which are equally necessary, or, more properly speaking, equal participants in the event. In fact, events are scientifically described by analyzing these participating factors and finding how they are related. (Kantor, 1959, p. 90)

This "expansion" of the field for investigation poses a myriad of challenges and implications for the clinician and requires a redefinition of the traditional role of the psychologist.

The Psychologist as Part of the Interbehavioral Field

In most settings, psychologists have functioned on a one-to-one therapist or counselor basis. This means of service delivery has proven often to be inadequate, particularly with the developmentally retarded population. This is because of a number of complex variables, including, but not limited to, insufficient financial resources, transportation and mobility problems, size of the service population, and the diversity of service needs often found within such systems. The role of psychologist as interbehaviorist provides alternatives to this traditional model.

The role of psychologist within a behavioral systems approach necessarily becomes that of a consultant, trainer, and systems analyst rather than a one-on-one therapist or counselor. Using the diverse behavioral technologies, psychologists travel within the community of the individuals being served to group and foster-care homes, workshops, and schools, thereby becoming an integral part of the support system of the individual. At the systems level, through interactions with the staff structure, procedures employed by the psychologist stand a better chance of lasting once the psychologist's formal involvement is faded out. This is because training the staff, rather than just the client, allows for staff to provide ongoing consistency of interactions not only with the target client but also with other clients under their charge who may be exhibiting similar behaviors.

A brief outline of the duties and responsibilities of the psychologist as interbehaviorist may help to clarify this new role. In addition to providing staff training for homes, schools, and workshops, the psychologist provides what may be viewed as "traditional" services (for example, testing). But the manner in which these duties are fulfilled follows the perspective of field behaviorism. Such duties of the psychologist fall within three major areas: testing and assessment, member of interdisciplinary team, and addressing (treating) problem behaviors.

First consider the area of testing and assessment. Although valid objections have been documented concerning the use of "intelligence" tests (Morgenstern, 1983), it must be recognized that mental health systems still require such testing on a periodic basis (Nelson, 1980). Under this imperative, behaviorally trained psychologists have managed to integrate traditional psychometry with methodologies of behavioral assessment. Psychologists deemphasize the importance of standardized IQ test scores and instead stress the objectively demonstrated relevance of providing a detailed and comprehensive adaptive skills assessment. This essentially consists of descriptive observations of those environmental factors interacting within the client's field (Leland, 1983; Rojahn & Schroeder, 1983).

Second, the psychologist performs an integral function as a member of an interdisciplinary treatment team. Psychologists determine and prepare short- and long-range goals and objectives for the client's achievement. The psychologist also performs an exhaustive adaptive skills assessment, defining the next steps in habilitative treatment, and writing concrete, operationally defined goals with specific consideration for the resources of the client and support staff during training.

Third, an important function of the psychologist is addressing problem behaviors. Again, however, this task need not be addressed in traditional ways. The psychologist might assess and define problem behaviors without centering solely upon the individual client. Instead, emphasis is placed on evaluation of the interactions of the client with staff and peers, as well as on the conditions and events that participate in the situation under observation. This is a major distinction from the methodologies employed for service delivery with this population. Particularly important here is the examination, observation, and targeting of the "complainant's" behavior.

The complainant is viewed as an integral part of the system and often becomes identified as the "client." Frequently it is the complainant's behavior and interactions (particularly the complaining behavior) that is the target for intervention. Here perhaps is the best demonstration of the new role of the psychologist—that of staff trainer rather than direct therapist in "treating" problem behaviors. This not only redefines the role of the psychologist (from that of primary therapist to staff trainer) but also redefines who the identified client is. The shift is from the traditionally defined individual service recipient to a broader perspective encompassing the client's peers and staff, their ongoing interactions, as well as the environing events which interact with their behaviors.

All of the duties outlined are aimed at assuring the maintenance of the clients within the community and their continued learning and development. Working with all levels of the system such as the home, schools, and community helps to ensure consistency of operations and continuity of care. The result is a psychological service delivery system which is *proactive* in that it functions to prevent the onset of problems or crises by training staff to identify needs before problems develop and *constructive* in that it emphasizes the need to refine or develop behavioral repertoires of the identified clients rather than to employ more traditionally oriented eliminative approaches.

The focus here is upon the system, not the individual. Examined are the client's behaviors across a variety of settings and conditions, the behaviors of the complainants, and other components of the total system. It must be noted that the psychologist working from this perspective is not merely an observer of behavior; he or she also is an integral participant in the system. Psychologists become involved in a case following the referral of problem behaviors. They also intervene in the system to construct the most effective support systems which prevent the onset and consequent referral of additional problems for correction.

Other Issues in Clinical Application

The interbehavioral perspective necessarily defines the type of precedures to be constructional rather than eliminative (Delprato, 1981; Goldiamond, 1974). While the two approaches are not always mutually exclusive, the emphasis upon constructing new behavioral repertoires is different from solely eliminating problem behaviors. This emphasis is integral in the effective and efficient delivery of psychological services within a behavioral systems framework. Constructional methodologies allow the therapist to avoid what in traditional terms is referred to as "symptom substitution." Using only eliminative procedures, it is not surprising to find that the individual may decrease a particular inappropriate behavior and instead engage in other behaviors equally inappropriate. The direction provided by constructional methodologies is in assisting the therapist to avoid such setbacks by initiating from the beginning of the planned intervention a methodology that teaches alternative or replacement behaviors to the problem behaviors. This does not leave to chance or trial and error that the client will exhibit "desirable" behaviors.

Additionally, presenting complaints (problem behaviors) are analyzed not as maladaptations to be overcome or eliminated but as adaptions made by an individual to particular circumstances. Adaptations of behavior thus are appropriate or inappropriate for the context, and they are concordant with the individual's interbehavioral history. Consequently, the therapist using constructional methodologies will refer to appropriate versus inappropriate behaviors (as socially defined) rather than to adaptive versus maladaptive behaviors. Inappropriate behaviors are examined within a broader perspective to determine events, individuals, and conditions which contribute to observed patterns of interaction; this also includes identifying where and in what manner the methodology for intervention should occur.

Emphasis is also placed upon working with the client and significant others (staff and care providers) within their natural environments and not in contrived laboratory-like settings to either observe, train, or intervene. Structuring contingencies that can be implemented in naturalistic settings is an important factor both in increasing the probability of initial intervention success and in the maintenance of behavioral changes over time. Two common problems seen in natural environment interventions require redefinition within this perspective: generalization and behavior compliance.

First, the issue of generalization as addressed in traditional behavioral systems is treated quite differently from an interbehavioral perspective. Rather than assuming there is generalization of behaviors from one setting to another as in conventional approaches, the interbehavioral systems approach actively examines various support variables across all settings; no setting is considered distinct but rather is interdependent upon all the past and potential settings in which the individual behaves. Hence, generalization fades as an issue.

Practitioners are frequently confronted by a second issue, that of noncompliance to treatment plans and recommendations. Within the systems perspective, compliance or noncompliance can no longer be viewed as an issue in the traditional sense. Interbehaviorally, noncompliance means a failure, but not in the sense of the client or staff failing to carry out or practice devised treatment strategies. It is instead the failure of practitioners to accurately identify and detail the variables that contribute to the maintenance of observed behaviors and interactions involving the client. Viewed in this manner, noncompliance encompasses the client's behaviors and interactions and also interactions of the psychologist in the system. Hence, the issue of compliance and noncompliance becomes more complex clinically but well-defined practically.

A similar issue is that of the use of medication to ''control'' behavior. Again, following a constructive approach, the attempt is to alleviate the use of medication as a mechanism for behavior control. Work in this area is twofold. First, through a network with other service providers within this system (including physicians, nurses, and psychiatrists) psychologists can demonstrate the effectiveness of behavior-change procedures over drug therapies. The attempt is not only to prevent the prescription of unneeded medication but also to reduce prolonged uses of prescribed medicines, which over extended periods of administration produce adverse and irreversible effects (e.g., tardive dyskinesia). This is consistent both with the previously outlined training role of the psychologist and with the constructional emphasis upon the acquisition and demonstration of ''new'' behavioral repertoires. Alternatives to medication frequently involve staff training to assure the consistency and appropriateness of interactions and the promotion and maintenance of appropriate behaviors by the client. The emphasis also is on prevention and correction of medically based disorders initially cited as responsible for the prescription.

A Case Study

A case example may help to illustrate and clarify the procedures employed by the interbehavioral psychologist working with the developmentally retarded population.

Client History

The client was a thirty-year-old male classified as functioning within the moderate range of mental retardation and adaptive impairment. He resided in a twelve-bed group home in an urban community. At the time of referral, he was participating in a sheltered workshop/day activity program five days per week where he performed both paid and mock work and attended various "classes," such as arts and crafts. The client was independently ambulatory with functional vision and hearing. His speech was extremely rapid and repetitive. He performed basic self-care activities when they were initiated by verbal prompts. Supervision was required in areas of community living skills (such as use of money, community travel, food preparation, time identification, survival signs, and so on).

Referral "Problem," Assessment, and Goals

The referral identified the client's problem behavior within the workshop setting as compulsive handwashing. As a result of interviewing workshop staff, the psychologist learned that the client was consistently out of his seat/work area for prolonged durations of time (one-half to one-hour intervals) and could usually be found in one of the restrooms of the shop. From a systems perspective, the problem was redefined as staff being unable to determine the location of the client consistently throughout the work day, requiring male staff (already few in number) to search the large, multilevel workshop structure to locate the client (a very time-consuming task). The psychologist also noted that although the client was always found in a bathroom washing his hands, this behavior (given the location) was not an inappropriate activity for the client. Assessment revealed that the client typically requested permission to leave his work/class area and received a "pass" to venture into other building areas (restrooms) along with verbal instructions to return within a specified time period (e.g., fifteen minutes). It was noteworthy that behavioral assessment revealed that the client did not (a) identify time even to within hour intervals (let alone minutes) and (b) own or wear a watch.

The interbehavioral perspective suggests several considerations at the point of assessment in the present case. Examination and review of all environing conditions were undertaken. These conditions included but were not limited to the current environmental setting, the behavior of the client, the skills of the client, the verbal/physical reports of the complainants, the workshop schedule, the staff involved in an ongoing/daily basis with the client, and the social-political exigencies of the system. The complainant became the client for services. And the environing conditions noted above were systematized in order to develop treatment goals and criteria for outcome success.

The goal for the "client" was not, as traditional behavior plans might suggest, the termination of compulsive handwashing behavior. Instead, following a proactive and constructive format, the goal was for the client to remain within his work area at appropriate times of the day and to return from his breaks and lunch hour within a specified time period. Concurrent with this goal were secondary goals for the client to increase his current take-home pay (which was usually between $0 and $0.50) and to learn to identify time.

Given workshop staffing limitations and the size of the workshop facility, the program to be implemented focused on the use of natural reinforcers for the client within the workshop setting, such as staff attention and verbal praise for appropriate behavior. Staff were no longer to conduct massive "manhunts" for the client throughout the workshop or utilize the paging system to call for the client. All periods of the day were to be constructed by staff to promote the client's return to his appropriate place within specified time periods.

Intervention

The above considerations led to the intervention program. A staff person was assigned to greet the client upon his entry to the workshop and accompany him to his work area. When the client arrived at his work station, he was praised and given a timer. When the client requested a break or when regularly scheduled breaks or the lunch hour occurred, staff set the client's timer for the designated time period (e.g., fifteen to forty-five minutes). The initial assessment revealed that staff frequently accompanied the client on his breaks. Therefore, in the first stage of intervention, a staff member accompanied the client's return to his work area in response to the auditory cue that occurred at the end of the timed interval. The presence of the staff was quickly faded so that the client soon used the timer cue as a discriminative stimulus to return to his work area independently. Upon arrival at the work area "on his own," the client was verbally praised for his prompt return. Within one week of the implementation of this program, the client was documented to be in his seat at appropriate times and to return from breaks within specified time periods at a frequency of 90 to 100 percent.

A documentation system for the intervention was established to provide data for the therapist and serve as an alteration of field factors designed to increase the likelihood that staff would perform in accordance with the program (i.e., comply with treatment recommendations). Measures included the duration of client breaks, frequency of client's timely return to his work station, frequency of staff praise or reinforcement of the client for appropriate behavior, number of requests made by client for unscheduled breaks, money earned by client, and number of breaks taken by client (scheduled and unscheduled) on a daily basis.

The above example highlights the techniques of the interbehavioral psychologist by illustrating how they function as a staff trainer rather than a one-on-one therapist, perform initial assessments of problem situations including the use of multiple response patterns and measures, redefine the target for intervention by viewing the complainant as the client, utilize constructive methodologies in treatment situations, design and use multiple measures for data collection, and act in a proactive fashion in that intervention occurred prior to the onset of a crisis situation thus averting the loss of the client's placement in an appropriate day program.

Conclusions

This chapter provides a general overview of the theoretical and technological aspects of a community-based service to developmentally retarded clients. In summary, the role of the psychologist is integral as a participant within the service delivery system of this client population. By impacting at the systems level, the psychologist (acting as a consultant) not only assures the delivery of effective behaviorally based services but also provides for the most efficient and economical means to alter interrelated problems dealing with staff and service structures. Looking ahead somewhat, advancement of the interbehavioral or systems approach for developmentally disabled populations may well promise a serious reassessment of goals, objectives, and values underlying the work of professionals in this area.

References

Berkson, G. 1978. Social ecology and ethology of mental retardation. In G. P. Sackett (Ed.), *Observing behavior: Theory and applications in mental retardation*, vol. 1. Baltimore: University Park Press, pp. 403–9.

Delprato, D. J. 1981. The constructional approach to behavioral modification. *Journal of Behavior Therapy and Experimental Psychiatry*, 12: 49–55.

Delprato, D. J. 1983, May. *Interacting response patterns: Contributions to constructional clinical behavioral intervention*. Paper presented at the meeting of the Association for Behavior Analysis, Milwaukee, Wisconsin.

Goldiamond, I. 1974. Toward a constructional approach to social problems. *Behaviorism* 2: 1–84.

Janicki, M. P., P. J. Castellani, and R. G. Norris. 1983. Organization and administration of service delivery systems. In J. Matson and J. Mulick (Eds.), *Handbook of mental retardation*. New York: Pergamon Press, pp. 3–23.

Kantor, J. R. 1924. *Principles of Psychology*, vol. 1. Granville, Ohio: Principia Press.

Kantor, J. R. 1959. *Interbehavioral psychology*. Bloomington, Ind.: Principia Press.

Kantor, J. R. 1968. Behaviorism in the history of psychology. *Psychological Record* 18: 151–66.

Kazdin, A. E. 1978. *History of behavior modification: Experimental foundations of contemporary research*. Baltimore: University Park Press.

Leland, H. 1983. Adaptive behavior scales. In J. Matson and J. Mulick (Eds.), *Handbook of mental retardation*. New York: Pergamon Press, pp. 215–25.

Matson, J. L. 1984. Psychotherapy with persons who are mentally retarded. *Mental Retardation* 22: 170–75.

Minuchin, S. 1974. *Families and family therapy*. Cambridge, Mass.: Harvard University Press.

Morgenstern, M. 1983. Standard intelligence tests and related assessment techniques. In J. Matson and J. Mulick (Eds.), *Handbook of mental retardation*. New York: Pergamon Press., pp. 201-14

Nelson, R. O. 1980. The use of intelligence tests within behavioral assesment. *Behavioral Assessment* 2: 417–23.

Nuffield, E. J. 1983. Psychotherapy. In J. Matson and J. Mulick (Eds.), *Handbook of mental retardation*. New York: Pergamon Press, pp. 351–68.

Patterson, G. R. 1975. *A social learning approach to family intervention*. Eugene, Ore.: Castalia Publishing Co.

Rojahn, J., and S. R. Schroeder. 1983. Behavioral asessment. In J. Matson and J. Mulick (Eds.), *Handbook of mental retardation*. New York: Pergamon Press, pp. 227–43.

Szasz, T. S. 1961. *The myth of mental illness*. New York: Harper & Row.

Whitman, T. L. and J. W. Scibak. 1981. Behavior modification research with the mentally retarded: Treatment and research perspectives. In J. L. Matson & J. R. McCartney (Eds.), *Handbook of behavior modification with the mentally retarded*. New York: Plenum, pp. 1–28.

13

Public Policy Research from a Field-Theory Perspective

Donna M. Cone

Public health policymakers seek to increase life expectancy and improve the quality of life of citizens within their political units. In North America and Western Europe, especially, public health practices have resulted in such dramatic benefits to humankind as the eradication of smallpox. Like public health in general, the field of public mental health attempts to prevent, or at least lessen, the negative effects of various disorders. Psychologists who pursue careers in public services administration, as opposed to those who select teaching, research, or private clinical practice, play key roles in the development and implementation of programs designed to promote the psychological well-being of the general populace.

Psychological or behavioral well-being results from larger and more complex *fields* of *interacting variables* than those fields that produce biological health. Hence, one might contrast the relatively straightforward relationship between drinking nonpasteurized milk and developing fever with the less clear relationship between child-rearing practices and neurotic behaviors of the child in adulthood. The successes of public policy interventions in clearly biological areas as opposed to areas involving many behavioral variables also reflect the relatively greater complexity of the latter fields. Witness the greater ease of protecting drinking water supplies from sewage as compared to persuading people to stop smoking cigarettes or to fasten their automobile seat belts.

In this chapter I will apply Kantor's interbehavioral perspective to the public policy issue of community living versus institutional living for mentally disabled individuals. Specifically, I will demonstrate how scientific principles can be used to answer the question of whether chronically mentally disabled individuals are better off living in small homes or in relatively larger hospital settings.

Interbehavioral Model Analyzing Public Policy

During his long and distinguished career, J. R. Kantor (1888–1984) stimulated students and colleagues alike to conduct experiments in all areas of psychology, using both human and nonhuman subjects. His most direct contributions to the behavioristic revolution are found in his stern critiques of psychology and the other sciences and in his careful exposition of the descriptive, or field study, approach.

Kantor's contributions were not fully appreciated by the laboratory-oriented psychology of midtwentieth-century North America. He chose not to conduct the usual kinds of research and not to direct a research laboratory staffed with devoted students. Kantor also preferred to publish without coauthors. His choice to minimize collaboration with fellow scientists and to rely primarily on his own observations and his own analyses of the published works of others put him out of the mainstream of behaviorism.

From his earliest major publication in the 1920s, the two-volume *Principles of Psychology*, Kantor held that complex human beings are capable of scientific analysis directly, without being reduced to reflexes. In the second volume of that work, Kantor (1926) devoted a chapter to the naturalistic analysis of such human activities as scientific behaviors, religious behaviors, and economic behaviors, among others. He also included a chapter on "abnormal reactions and psychopathic personalities." In the latter chapter, Kantor contrasted the approaches of psychologists and psychiatrists, noted the significant role of sociocultural factors in setting the standards by which behaviors are judged "abnormal" and argued that "the psychological study of abnormality calls for the inclusion of all exaggerations and singularities whatsoever" (p. 458).

An approach to the scientific study of complex human behaviors, which Kantor described in detail in two of his later books, seems to have been overlooked by clinicians and public policymakers alike. This approach, which is based on what Kantor called "remote observation," consists of an analysis of the observations of others in which the analyst plays the role of logician of science.

In the body of this chapter, I will demonstrate how this analysis can be used to address the question of whether public mental health policy should support community or institutional living arrangements for individuals with a condition of chronic mental disability. It will also become clear that such an analysis can be conducted prior to an experimental study of complex human behaviors to assist the scientist in designing the experiment. Why conduct an armchair analysis rather than a program evaluation study? The answer to this question has both practical and philosophical aspects.

Program Evaluations: Interbehavioral Considerations

Program evaluation studies of the effects of living arrangements on psychological adjustment, like all longitudinal studies, take a long time to complete.

Public policy shifts in this country occur over a relatively short time span, ranging from the four-year term of the U.S. president to the longer time it takes for the U.S. Congress to drift to the right or left or for the U.S. Supreme Court to become liberal or conservative.

A number of practical considerations apply, such as how long is long enough to make sure that optimal adjustment has occurred. In addition, it is difficult to find a group of subjects to follow that will remain in a given geographic area so that the community environment is relatively uniform and the individuals are available for follow-along assessments. The research team, or at least its leadership, must be committed to the project for years. The expense of conducting longitudinal studies is relatively high compared with other types of research. For example, the analysis of large amounts of data over time requires ready access to computers and the conducting of client assessments requires much professional staff time (Woolson, Tsuang, & Urban, 1980). In addition, as C. M. Harding and G. W. Brooks (1980, p. 274) note, "how to fully utilize the richness of the data, and . . . how to cope with early research decisions made . . . years ago, which affect current research efforts" constitute significant problems for the long-term follow-up study team.

A more significant point is that there is nothing to be gained by making thousands of observations of clients and measuring thousands of instances of their complex behaviors if the researcher does not apply a logic of science that allows the legitimate transformation of those data into a valid general finding.

Like other behaviorists, Kantor viewed the goals of psychology as understanding, prediction, and control. He described four generalized scientific procedures: direct observation, instrumental observation, transforming contacts (as when a chemist analyzes and synthesizes compounds), and remote observation (generalizing and analogizing) (Kantor, 1953, p. 16). This last procedure is most relevant to our present undertaking.

Kantor describes remote observations as "the most subtle forms of scientific activity," being "indirect and remote inferential operations" (1953, p. 16). The scientist's emphasis remains on "basic encounters with events" and while "the chain connecting the worker and the thing upon which he operates may consist of many links . . . it is characteristic of scientific work that the connection is rigidly maintained" (Kantor, 1953, p. 16).

In the *Logic of Modern Science*, Kantor states that "logic is the science of systems" and that "when the logician of science analyzes a scientific situation he is himself engaging in a scientific enterprise" (1953, p. 26). What a welcome contrast this is to the frequently heard disdain for "armchair scientists" who are viewed as behaving nonscientifically simply because they are not in a laboratory or open field setting observing behavioral events directly.

Kantor pictures the logician of science as developing a five-factor system: crude data (familiar objects, discoveries, syntheses), operations (investigative contacts with events), products (hypotheses, theories, laws), the thing and event matrix (both original and contrived), and cultural sources (folklore, scientific traditions) (1953, pp. 26–28). The subject matter for the logician of science is the work of the original investigator under the exact conditions that prevailed during the original research.

The work of logicians of science is primarily critical, or evaluative. They check for such things as appropriateness of the experimental design, correct usage of statistics, and validity of conclusions based on observed data. Of key importance is the use of the things and events as criteria to correct errors on the part of the original investigator. Kantor points out the essence of the logician of science's work as follows:

Scientists . . . operate in a middle ground between two constraining borders: on one side the immense domain of things, processes and events, including the scientist; on the other the cultural insititutions which influence his ways of thinking and his operational techniques. The logician's task is to estimate the relative proportion of findings the scientist derives from cultural and from event sources . . . if the ratio favors cultural influences, it is clear that the worker is misinterpreting his data. (1953, p. 26).

The cultural influences of which Kantor spoke are broadly defined to include both behavior and products of behavior. Cultural behavior included "every variety of interaction with things, persons and events" which are "all rooted in the biological process of self, family, and group maintenance" (1953, p. 45). Cultural behavior products are likewise ubiquitous, including rites, customs, and manners as well as tools, symbols, and institutions.

Kantor (1963) presented an advanced example of remote observation which he labeled "tertiary scientific level" or "historico-critical level" of psychological history as scientific method. At this level, the critic or analyst interbehaves with the historian who interbehaves with the original investigator. The illustration of this approach can easily be transformed to show the public policy maker as the analyst, the evaluator as the historian, the clinician as the primary observer, and the patient as the original subject of study (See Figure 13.1).

Materials from Kantor's *Interbehavioral Psychology* (1959) emphasize that the psychological event-field is dynamic and evolves across time. The development of behavioral adjustments across time is clearly of great importance in evaluating the effects of living arrangements on patients.

The Analysis

Step one of the historico-critical analysis would seem to be to select the work of one or more primary investigators and begin to evaluate it critically. However, there are two general points to be considered, each of which can profoundly shape the outcome of the logical analysis.

The first is the scientific method used by the original investigator(s). Mary Hesse (1980) and other contemporary philosphers of science have articulately pointed out the limitations of the traditional positivistic method used by most

Figure 13.1
Interbehavior of a Public Policymaker with a Reaction of an Evaluator

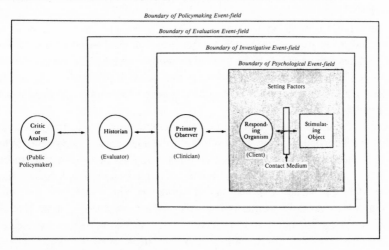

Source: J. R. Kantor, *The Scientific Evolution*
of Psychology, vol. 1 (Chicago: Principia Press, 1963).

modern Western scientists. Y. S. Lincoln and E. G. Guba (1985) have taken
these critiques seriously and developed the alternative pradigm of "naturalistic
inquiry" which they apply to the areas of education research and program evaluation, among others.

Like Kantor, Lincoln and Guba cite the impact of values on scientific activity.
Four major types of values which they list as having a direct impact are personal
values of the investigator (e.g., the choice of a problem); values inherent in the
chosen paradigm (e.g., a behavioristic versus a psychoanalytic one); values
inherent in the substantive theory used to guide the collection, analysis, and
interpretation of data (e.g., the positivistic assumption that the scientist seeks
truth); and general cultural values that characterize the society in which the
research occurs (e.g., the Third Reich's search for ways to breed a superior race)
(Lincoln & Guba, 1985, pp. 38, 174–77).

A self-examination by an analyst can shed light on how personal values and
the paradigm used by the analyst influence the selection and evaluation of the
reports of observations, hypotheses, and conclusions of others. Let me illustrate
how my own values and training can be expected to shape the outcome of my
analysis of living arrangements: I strongly value independence and self-sufficiency; I am an interbehaviorist and subscribe to a naturalistic, as opposed to a
positivistic, philosophy of science; I have invested the past eleven years of my
life in working to improve state institutions and to provide noninstitutional living
opportunities for mentally disabled persons; and I am politically liberal, inclined
toward civil activism, and I enjoy challenging authority. Given these self-ob-

servations, how likely am I to conclude that all chronically mentally disabled people are hopelessly ill and should live in centralized psychiatric hospital settings?

The second general point to be considered is the idiographic nature of the thing and event matrix. Inasmuch as each psychological event is unique, how can findings from one setting be applied to another setting? The reader will note that when Lincoln and Guba (1985) raise this question they are asking how the generalizing and analogizing of Kantor's remote observation approach can be legitimately realized.

Lincoln and Guba note that the person attempting the application must have sufficient knowledge about both settings to render a valid judgment. While Lincoln and Guba see it as impossible for the original investigators to specify all contexts to which their working hypotheses might be transferred, these authors do see it as a reasonable expectation that workers provide a sufficient description of the contextual field so that others may make a judgment of transferability (1985). A vital first question to be asked by the analyst is whether or not there is sufficient available information to judge the fit between the context already studied and that proposed to be explained or predicted by the previous findings.

Identification of Primary Investigations

Several recognized approaches to locating original studies and evaluations of studies are available to the analyst (Mountjoy & Sears, 1971; Mountjoy, 1974). The approach used must be specified since the representativeness and comprehensiveness of the sample used by the analyst will affect the conclusions reached.

I used three interrelated approaches in the present analysis. A mental health librarian searched the *Index Medicus* from 1980 to 1985, using the names of four investigators I had located during a preliminary literature search; I reviewed the articles she located and selected additional studies from their reference lists; I visited with two of the four investigators, C. M. Harding and M. T. Tsuang. For practical reasons, I have used only sources published in English. Five books and approximately 100 articles were reviewed.

These materials fell into the following topic groupings: (a) long-term follow-up studies; (b) studies on the definition of schizophrenia; (c) studies of variables predicting a positive outcome; (d) related studies, such as differential mortality rates in clients with differing diagnoses; (e) works that demonstrate the impact of long-term study results on clinical practice and evaluation. This last category is particularly interesting because it shows that at least two investigators, J. S. Strauss and Harding, have been led by the data to modify the traditional scientific approach. These modifications appear compatible with some major aspects of both Kantor's interbehavioral perspective and the naturalistic method of Lincoln and Guba.

Long-term Follow-up Studies

Two American and two European projects with catamnestic periods of at least twenty years were analyzed, together with one Canadian and three American projects that followed clients for shorter periods. All eight projects used a more or less traditional scientific approach in that large samples were analyzed using parametric statistics. Operational definitions were specified and care was taken to minimize bias by using blind techniques and interobserver-reliability checks. The projects are all fairly recent. (Readers interested in locating studies published prior to 1970 should see Stephens, 1978).

A. *The Iowa 500 Study.* Tsuang, R. F. Woolson, and J. A. Fleming (1979) and Tsuang and M. Dempsey (1979) describe a thirty- to forty-year follow-up field study of 610 patients admitted to the University of Iowa Psychiatric Hospital and 160 surgical patients admitted to the University General Hospital between 1934 and 1944. Of the 770 individuals studied, 200 persons had been diagnosed as schizophrenic; 325 suffered from affective disorders; 85 had both schizophrenia and affective disorders; and 160 psychiatric symptom-free surgical patients served as controls. Data were gathered from medical records and from telephone and face-to-face interviews with the patients and their close relatives. The Iowa Structured Psychiatric Interview (Tsuang, 1980) was used. A three-point scale of good, fair, and poor estimated outcome on four variables, marital, occupational, residential, and psychiatric status. (The reader will note that the selection of outcome measures clearly reflected cultural values in that, for example, it was judged a better outcome to be married than single and to be working than unemployed). Overall, the psychiatric patients had poorer status outcomes than the surgical controls and the schizophrenic patients faired significantly less well than those with affective disorders, with the 85 schizoaffective patients falling in between the other two psychiatric groups. Nevertheless, the schizophrenic patients received "good" ratings as follows: marital (21 percent), occupational (35 percent), residential (34 percent), and psychiatric (20 percent).

B. *The Bonn Study.* G. Huber, G. Gross, R. Schutter, and M. Linz (1980) studied between 1967 and 1973, 502 schizophrenic patients who had been admitted to the University Psychiatric Clinic of Bonn, Germany, between 1945 and 1959. Complete psychopathological remissions occurred in 22 percent of the patients, with 43 percent showing partial remission and 35 percent suffering chronic schizophrenic deficiencies. The determination of remission status involved an evaluation of social and occupational variables, among others.

C. *The Lausanne Investigation.* L. Ciompi (1980) reported on 289 schizophrenic patients over an observation period of thirty-seven years. These surviving individuals were part of an original group of 1,642 former patients of the University Psychiatric Clinic of Lausanne, Switzerland, who were less than sixty-five years old at first hospital admission and who had been born between 1873 and 1897. Documents were studied, a two-hour semistructured interview occurred in the client's home, and significant other people (for example, family members and physicians) were consulted. The investigators concluded that about three-fifths of the persons studied between 1964 and 1969 had either recovered or shown clear improvement. The average age of the 289 persons was over seventy-five years and a "calming" effect of age on symptomatology was noted. Fifty-six percent were living outside psychiatric hospitals; more than half were in good physical health; 15 percent were fully employed, while 37 percent worked part-time; and 17 percent were married.

D. *The Vermont Longitudinal Research Project.* C. M. Harding (1984) and Harding, G. W. Brooks, T. Ashikaga, J. S. Strauss, and P. D. Landerl (in press) provide recent descriptions of a thirty-year-long study of chronic, state hospital patients. When selected for a rehabilitation program in 1955, the patients were "middle-aged, poorly educated, mostly single, lower class individuals . . . [with] an average of 10 years disability, and six years continuous hospitalization" (Chittick, Brooks, Irons, & Deane, 1961, p. 29). Two hundred sixty-nine of these patients were studied in the early 1960s and it was found that about two-thirds of them were living outside the hospital with an array of support services (Daum, Brooks, & Albee, 1977). In the mid–1970s, 89 percent of the original cohort was located and an assessment of a stratified subset of thirty-eight persons showed their continuing ability to live in community settings (Daum, et al., 1977). In 1982, ninety-seven percent of the cohort was again located or accounted for, yielding a total of 149 persons to assess with structured interviews (Harding, et al., in press). Ninety-five percent were currently living in the community and fifty-four percent were single.

A modified sociogram was consructed and used to determine just how socially isolated was this group of older chronic patients (fifty-seven percent were then over the age of sixty). Forty-five percent had one or more close or rather close friends and sixty-seven percent met with friends at least every week or two. Field observations revealed three basic styles of interpersonal relationships: the "niche group," for whom specific living and/or working situations had evolved wherein they thrived; the "loners," who had deliberately chosen to live alone and work intermittently; and the "self-regulators," who did not seem to develop close friends but rather carefully controlled and limited social contacts. Harding (1984) reported the results of blindly rediagnosing the 269 original cohort members using the DSM III (APA, 1980) process. Eighty-two of the 118 subjects who met the DSM III criteria for a schizophrenia diagnosis were interviewed twice; relatives and significant others were interviewed; and hospital records were reviewed. One-half to two-thirds of these people had "achieved much fuller lives than had been expected" (Harding, 1984, p. 52). Sixty percent of the subjects fell into the category of "good functioning" on the Global Assessment Scale (Endicott, Spitzer, Fleiss, & Cohen, 1976), with the remaining 40 percent in "fair functioning." Of those in the "good" category, 53 percent were single and 24 percent were fully employed, as compared to 74 percent single and 3 percent (one person) fully employed in the "fair" category.

E. *Four Shorter-Term Studies.* D. M. Engelhardt, B. Rosen, J. Feldman,

J. Z. Engelhardt, and P. Cohen (1982) reported on the fifteen-year hospitalization course of 646 chronic schizophrenic patients, aged eighteen to forty-five, referred to the Psychopharmacology Treatment and Research Clinic of the Kings County Hospital Center in Brooklyn, New York, between 1958 and 1963. Twenty-one percent had never been hospitalized, twenty-two percent had had crisis admissions only, and fifty-seven percent had had long-term psychiatric hospitalization. During the fifteen years reviewed, sixty-nine percent of the group was hospitalized at least once. Those with no previous hosptialization were less likely to be hospitalized than the crisis admissions who, in turn, were less likely to be hospitalized than patients with a history of long-term hospitalization. The authors concluded that with phenothiazine therapy, fully forty-one percent of schizophrenics could be maintained on an outpatient basis. The remaining individuals needed repeated, and sometimes fairly long-term, access to inpatient treatment.

G. Gardos, J. O. Cole, and R. A. LaBrie (1982) reported a twelve-year follow-up study of 90 of 124 chronic schizophrenic patients who comprised the Boston State Hospital cohort of a collaborative study of high-dose chlorpromazine therapy. In 1977 interviews were conducted using the Global Assessment Scale (Endicott, et al., 1976) and the Psychiatrist's Global Rating of Illness Scale. Twenty-three percent of the 90 individuals were hospitalized, with 39 percent in nursing homes, 6 percent with families, 13 percent in family care settings, 14 percent in cooperative apartments, and 5 percent in lodgings. Severity of illness ratings and Global Assessment Scale scores were significantly different when the hospitalized group was compared with the groups living most independently (for example, in apartments and lodgings). Those living in the least restrictive community settings were less severely ill and better adjusted. The authors concluded that "those patients who were discharged into the community during the first wave of the deinstitutionalization drive of the 1960s have shown marked and significant improvement over 12 years"(p. 984).

R. C. Bland, J. H. Parker, and H. Orn (1976) reported a ten-year study of eighty-eight of ninety-two schizophrenic patients first admitted to the Alberta Hospital in Ponoka, Canada, in 1963. A semistructured interview was used to gather various social, economic, and psychiatric outcome data from the patients and significant others. At follow-up, fifty-eight percent were adjudged recovered from psychiatric symptoms, and another nine percent showed periodic, mild symptoms; thirty-five percent had made good social adjustments and thirty-four percent fair social adjustments; fifty-one percent held regular jobs and another eighteen percent worked fairly regularly; forty-nine percent were single. Only eight percent of the patients were unremittingly hospitalized; seventy-five percent had zero, one, or two hospital readmissions; fifty-six percent had had no care from a psychiatrist during the two years preceding the survey; and sixty-two percent were taking medication for psychiatric conditions. The authors contribute their positive findings to "short initial hospitalization, almost universal use of phenothiazines, use of developing community services (social and psychiatric), and generally good economic conditions" (p. 949).

G. E. Vaillant (1978) reported following for an average of ten years, fifty-one schizophrenic patients who were admitted to the Massachusetts Mental Health Center between 1959 and 1962 and who achieved full remission of psychiatric symptoms. Medical records indicated that twenty of the patients (40 percent) relapsed and spent an average of 25 percent of the follow-up period hospitalized. Except for brief periods of relapse in a few cases, the remaining thirty-one (60 percent) maintained symptom remission. Twenty-one of these thirty-one people were interviewed at least ten years after first admission. Each appeared nonschizophrenic, none was on phenothiazine therapy, and all maintained employment and good social functioning.

Summary. Taken as a whole, these eight follow-up studies suggest that with the use of modern therapeutic interventions, both psychiatric and social, the majority of chronic schizophrenic patients do get better and many recover completely. This overall conclusion derives from a sampling of studies that included various lengths of follow-up, both rural and urban settings in Europe and North America, and patients ranging in age from young adulthood to old age. In a selective review of follow-up studies, Tsuang emphasized individual variability in the course of schizophrenia and concluded that "on the average, 25% of schizophrenics recover, 50% remain behaviorally impaired, and 25% do not recover" (1982, p. 203).

To public policymakers, such general group findings appear adequate to justify a treatment system that emphasizes community-based living and supportive services and, at the same time, contains a crisis intervention capability, as well as psychiatric hospital services for the minority of persons who intermittently need the more protected setting. Indeed, given the reliable epidemiological estimate that 0.5 percent to 3.0 percent of the population exhibits the condition of schizophrenia at any given time (Strauss & Carpenter, 1981) policymakers have the data needed to determine the size of each treatment system component for the political unit within their purview.

While the state of affairs is desirable from a systems perspective, it offers little direction for the assignment of individuals to loci within the treatment system. Given a value system that lauds self-sufficiency, economic productivity, and the ability to escape the stigmatization of being labeled "mentally ill," what do the data tell the policymaker and clinician about increasing the number of people who recover from functional psychoses?

Predicting Good Outcomes

By comparing the intake records of fifty schizophrenic patients displaying good outcome after five years with those of fifty patients who showed poor outcome, J. H. Stephens, C. Astrup, and J. C. Mangrum (1966) discovered eleven factors that differentiated between the two groups. Four factors were significant ($p<.01$): depressive, not schizoid, guilt, and confusion. Three factors were significant at $p<.05$ level: no low IQ, no emotional blunting, and no schizophrenic heredity. Among the forty-three factors that did not differentiate between the two groups were age, sex, and a variety of behaviors generally used to diagnose subtypes of schizophrenia (e.g., paranoid delusions).

As Vaillant (1978) pointed out, the discovery of such seeming predictors led researchers to believe that persons achieving full remission must be qualitatively different from those who remain chronically disabled. Two basic hypotheses were developed to explain this alleged difference, one related to etiology and the other to diagnosis. Etiologically, chronic schizophrenia was believed to be genetically based while remitting schizophrenia was seen as psychogenic in origin; diagnostically, various attempts were made to refine procedures so that only instances of "true" or "core" schizophrenia received that diagnostic label. Among the well-known latter approaches are Langfeldt's schizophreniform diagnosis for those who show remission and the evolution of the DSM III diagnostic criteria. In his 1978 study of Massachusetts patients, Vaillant failed to find support for there being two types of schizophrenia and suggested that "remission and diagnosis can be thought of as two different dimensions of psychosis" (p. 83).

Strauss and Carpenter (1974a) directly tested the hypothesis that different diagnostic methods would lead to improved outcome predictions. In introducing this study, the authors cited some historical and cultural variables that have shaped thinking about diagnosis and outcome. In the late nineteenth century, Emil Kraeplin used poor prognosis as a validating criterion for dementia praecox. When Eugen Bleuler broadened this diagnostic category and renamed it schizophrenia he emphasized even more this poor outcome factor. In the United States, many psychiatrists followed Adolph Meyer's lead and abandoned outcome as a validity criterion while in Europe the opposite occurred, with many psychiatrists insisting that a patient who recovered could not be a true schizophrenic. Strauss and Carpenter concluded that "much of the evidence for poor outcome arises from the diagnosis not being given until after it is clear that the patient has a chronic disorder, suggesting that the poor prognosis of schizophrenia may not be so much a validity criterion as a tautology that chronic patients are chronic" (1974a, p. 430). Using methodological controls absent in earlier studies, Strauss and Carpenter (1974a) compared several diagnostic systems, including that of Langfeldt, in order to evaluate any relationship between characteristic symptoms and outcome. No such relationship was demonstrated.

Using a cohort of the WHO (World Health Organization) International Pilot Study of Schizophrenia as subjects, Strauss and Carpenter (1974b) discovered three key predictor variables for two-year outcome. Employment history predicted employment outcome, social history predicted social outcome, and established chronicity of illness (previous hospitalizations) predicted outcome in all areas. They suggested that "outcome is not a single process but it is comprised of several semi-independent processes best conceptualized as open-linked systems" (p. 37). In 1977, Strauss and Carpenter found that five-year follow-up, key predictors were still previous social contacts, previous employment, and previous hospitalization, plus a new one, treatment facilities. The easiest variable to measure, hospitalization, had the lowest correlation with the other outcome variables. Level of social relationships prior to initial evaluation was a significant predictor of all outcome variables at five-year follow-up.

In a study of ex-mental patients living in a large Manhattan hotel, C. I. Cohen and J. Sokolovsky (1978) provided data to support the importance of current social relationships in maintaining good outcome. They found that while schizophrenics have fewer social linkages than do nonpsychotics, even the most impaired schizophrenics are not totally isolated. Among schizophrenics the social network varied by size, complexity, directionality, and interconnectedness. Rehospitalization was a function of degree of psychopathology and social network size.

Four studies suggest additional variables that may affect predicted outcome. A. F. Fontana and B. N. Dowds (1975) noted the importance of the perspective of the evaluator when they demonstrated that significant others tend to describe patients as less well adjusted than the patients themselves in areas of employment, organizational participation, and alcohol abuse, but not in symptomatology and social involvement. Significant others were again implicated by the finding of C. E. Vaughan and J. P. Leff (1976) that expressed emotion of relatives (number of critical comments made when discussing the patient and his or her illness, hostility, and marked emotional overinvolvement) is associated with relapse independently of all other social and clinical factors studied.

Therapist characteristics were shown differentially to affect patient outcome when schizophrenics were treated by drugs alone and by psychotherapy plus drugs, but not by electroconvulsive shock therapy, psychotherapy alone, or milieu (a control where none of the other four treatments was used) (Tuma, May, Yale, & Forsythe, 1978). The initial two-year follow-up of the WHO International Pilot Study of Schizophrenia of 1,202 patients in nine countries found that patients in developing countries had better outcomes than patients in developed countries (58 percent of Nigerian patients and 47 percent of Indian patients were symptom-free, as compared with 8 percent of Danish patients and 1 percent of Russian patients) (Tsuang, 1982).

The predictor variables discussed above were discovered in studies of formerly institutionalized schizophrenic patients. What about the increasingly large numbers of chronically mentally ill persons who have had only brief or no psychiatric hospitalization? H. R. Lamb and V. Goertzel (1977) studied a sample of ninety-nine community residents who were eighteen to sixty-four years old selected from those with functional psychotic diagnosis who received Supplemental Security Income (SSI) in San Mateo, California. Only 4 percent had been hospitalized in a state hospital in the previous two years while thirty-two percent had spent time in local mental hospitals, both public and private, during that time. Twenty-three persons received no outpatient services, while thirty used private-sector services only; twenty-seven used public-sector services only and nineteen used a combination of public and private outpatient services. Thirty-six percent had no medications prescribed, while fifty percent had major psychotropic drugs prescribed and 13 percent had minor tranquilizers and antidepressants prescribed. Fifty-six percent of the sample had no structured employment activity. More than two-thirds lived either with their families or independently. The authors discussed an impression they had that many patients had opted for a relatively isolated life that minimized anxiety, thus allowing them to remain in the community. While such isolation and inactivity is viewed as regressive by most mental health professionals, Lamb and Goertzel saw a deliberate choice of this option as a patient's prerogative. They concluded with an emphasis on the importance of SSI in maintaining individuals outside state hospitals.

The widely respected authority on treatment and living arrangements for mentally diabled persons, Leona Bachrach (1980), listed eight principles that she believed constitute effective program design for chronic patients: chronic patients targeted, linkage with other resources, functional integrity, individually tailored treatment, cultural relevance and specificity, specially trained staff, hospital liaison, and internal evaluation. She stressed that effective programs are effective not only because they have these eight characteristics but because they acknowledge that chronic mental patients "have severe and recurrent problems, that they are often functionally impaired and in need of assistance in gaining access to the most basic of life's entitlements, and, most of all, that their individuality is of greater significance in effective treatment than any categorical label" (p. 1026).

The importance of these idiosyncratic data, which present themselves as irritating exceptions to the general theories and laws which nomothetic researchers seek, has been recognized by both Strauss and Harding and their coworkers. It is instructive to trace the evolution of their research away from the traditional epidemiological approach to an approach that focuses on the individual client.

Individual Field Models

C. M. Daum, G. W. Brooks, and G. W. Albee (1977) questioned the usual procedure of assigning on outcome scales higher scores to married clients than to unmarried ones. They noted that ex-patients frequently marry ex-patients and, in all cases observed in this study, the couple functioned less well than the unmarried clients.

J. S. Strauss and H. Hafez (1981) built the case that traditional large-sample (quantitative) studies should be complemented by the systematic development of clinical intuition in the clinical setting (qualitative). Responding to anecdotal material from schizophrenic patients, Strauss, L. Loevsky, W. Glazer, and P. Leaf (1981) demonstrated this qualitative approach by analyzing symptoms, the patient's work situation and the relationship between the two. A systems model emerged in which certain aspects of the patient's work affected certain aspects of his or her symptomatology.

Strauss and Glazer (1982) identified four aspects of chronicity (chronic symptoms; chronic social and occupational dysfunction; chronic treatment; chronic attitude or acceptance of being permanently disabled or bizarre) in an attempt to focus on individual clients and their strengths. In fact, few clients display all aspects of chronicity at any given time and many function very well in some important life areas while still displaying some aspects of chronicity. The authors focused on treatment intensity, noting that some patients are ready for intensive treatment approaches while others are not, and this may change over time for the individual. The clue that a patient is ready for intensive intervention seems to be a lessening of the chronic attitude.

A. Breir and Strauss (1983) documented with twenty chronically ill patients the ability of individuals to control their own psychiatric symptoms. In a dramatic example of the importance of listening to the client and following one's clinical intuition, the authors discovered that seventeen of the twenty patients interviewed employed three major kinds of self-control techniques: self-instruction, decreased involvement in activity, and increased involvement in activity. The seventeen self-controllers, as contrasted with the three clients who did not control their own symptoms, heeded early signs of psychotic behaviors in themselves and took corrective action.

Strauss, Hafez, Lieberman, and Harding (1985) collected data from twenty-eight patients over a two-year period following hospital discharge. By interviewing them bimonthly in the first year and again at the end of the second year, these authors obtained a finer-grain picture of the course of functional psychiatric disorders than was previously available. They discovered eight longitudinal principles in the two categories of longitudinal patterns and individual-environment interactions. Recovery was not linear; indeed, clearly definable patterns emerged with periods of moratorium, change points, and ceilings. Clients were found to be active participants in their recovery and it was possible to ferret out a variety of environmental factors (family behaviors and expectations, stressful events, and so on) which shaped the individual's posthospitalization course.

Harding and Strauss (in press) conclude that the course of schizophrenia "needs to be assessed across contexts, and across individual components of a developing person. Course appears to be shaped by the person-environment interaction and the goodness of fit between these two" (p. 12). This conclusion is clearly compatible with Kantor's interbehavioral model. The approach used by Strauss, Harding, and their coworkers is basically the case-report method advocated by Lincoln and Guba (1985).

The conclusions that present themselves to the idiographic (or qualitative) researcher are markedly different from those discovered by the nomothetic (or quantitative) researcher. Gareth Morgan (1983) observed that true scientists include in their frame of reference not only the object under study, but also the protocol and technique through which the object becomes meaningful. The scientist and the methods used all remain interdependent and in constant motion.

The interaction Development Model which Strauss, Harding, and their coworkers are developing holds clear implications for the individualized treatment of chronically mentally disabled persons. It also contributes new data to our science, data which are authentic, naturalistic, and nonreductionistic, as Kantor envisioned in his earliest consideration of complex human behaviors over sixty years ago.

Conclusions and Future Considerations

The remote observation approach has been applied to the leading long- and short-term studies that followed schizophrenic patients after discharge from psychiatric hospitals. When analyzed by an observer who admits to holding democratic, highly moral values characteristic of many contemporary public policymakers, these studies strongly suggest that small, community living arrangements are superior to large, centralized institutions. In the interest of meeting the needs of those clients who from time to time require the increased protection of a hospital setting, a continuum of services from highly restrictive to relatively nonrestrictive seems desirable.

Most of the pesons whose progress was followed after discharge from hospitals had long histories of institutionalization. Many came of age in an institution, never realizing their potential for independence. Remotivation of these individuals whose hopes and desires had been smothered by decades of hospitalization became the job of small, specialized residential settings. Case management programs, medication, psychotherapy, and rehabilitation have evolved as the professional support for community living.

Recently there has emerged a new generation of persons disabled by mental illness for whom long-term institutionalization is neither appropriate nor available. Their service needs are difficult to define and provide for. These are the young adults who might or might not be willing to accept the help currently available through the network of community mental health agencies.

The first generation of persons with severe mental illness who will never face institutional care provide special challenges for mental health planners and human service providers. Services need to be restructured and further developed to help meet identified needs rather than attempting to mold the new generation into an older, less appropriate service spectrum.

To further describe the new generation of mental health consumers, one need only look at the larger population of younger people. For most, the goals of independence, a good job, a new place to live, decent clothing, and enough money are of key importance. Sexuality is an important factor. For some, the use of alcohol and other drugs can be an issue. The role of being disabled and dependent is both unfitting and unwanted. The clinical diagnosis for the younger person is often the same as that applied to the deinstitutionalized generation—schizophrenia, manic-depressive illness, personality disorder—yet psychodiagnostic categories do little to aid in planning for effective interventions.

Who then speaks for the new generation of disabled people? Fortunately, among others, they themselves do. Consumer groups are being organized and are becoming active on several fronts, such as public relations efforts to extinguish myths about mentally ill people and attempts to outlaw electroconvulsive shock therapy.

There is no doubt that the young consumer often makes demands on the service delivery system that are difficult to address: crises that arise in the middle of the night, confounding involvement with drugs and alcohol, a basic unwillingness to play by rules that seem restrictive and unfair, and a suspiciousness of medications that might ameliorate some of their more distressing symptoms. These demands call for services not universally available, such as temporary or crisis housing, support and assistance outside an office setting, vocational programming that involves more than "make work" and minimum wages.

Clearly these young adults will need a spectrum of residential services from supervised apartments through more diverse and imaginative group homes and the involvement of critical groups in service design and implementation. Unlike many of their predecessors, these clients will be able to critique their services and contribute positively to their improvement.

The best assistance that professionals and public policymakers can give to all mentally disabled people is to be aware of the cultural variables that shape behavior, to be concerned for individual needs and strengths, and to be open to new patterns emerging from the event-field.

References

American Psychiatric Association. 1980. *Diagnostic and statistical manual III*. Washington, D.C.: APA.

Bachrach, L. 1980. Overview: Model programs for chronic mental patients. *American Journal of Psychiatry* 137: 1023–31.

Bland, R. C., J. H. Parker, and H. Orn. 1976. Prognosis in schizophrenia: A ten-year follow-up of first admissions. *Archives of General Psychiatry* 33: 949-54.

Breir, A., and J. S. Strauss. 1983. Self-control in psychotic disorders. *Archives of General Psychiatry* 40: 1141–45.

Chittick, R. A., G. W. Brooks, F. A. Irons, and W. N. Deane. 1961. *The Vermont story*. Burlington, Vt.: Queen City Printers.

Ciompi, L. 1980. Catamnestic long-term study on the course of life and aging of schizophrenics. *Schizophrenia Bulletin* 6: 606–18.

Cohen, C. I., and J. Sokolovsky. 1978. Schizophrenia and social networks: Expatients in the inner city. *Schizophrenia Bulletin* 4: 546–60.

Daum, C. M., G. W. Brooks, and G. W. Albee. 1977. Twenty-year follow-up of 253 schizophrenic patients originally selected for chronic disability: Pilot study. *Psychiatric Journal of the Unviersity of Ottawa* 2: 129–32.

Endicott, J., R. L. Spitzer, J. L. Fleiss, and J. Cohen. 1976. The Global Assessment Scale: A procedure for measuring overall severity of psychiatric disturbance. *Archives of General Psychiatry* 33: 766–71.

Englehardt, D. M., B. Rosen, J. Feldman, J. Z. Engelhardt, and P. Cohen. 1982. A 15-

year followup of 646 schizophrenic outpatients. *Schizophrenia Bulletin* 8: 493–503.

Fontana, A. F., and B. N. Dowds. 1975. Assessing treatment outcome, I. Adjustment in the community. *Journal of Nervous and Mental Disease* 161: 221–30.

Gardos, G., J. O. Cole, and R. A. LaBrie. 1982. A 12-year follow-up study of chronic schizophrenics. *Hospital and Community Psychiatry* 33: 983–84.

Harding, C. M. 1984. *Long-term outcome functioning of subjects rediagnosed as meeting the DSM III criteria for schizophrenia.* Unpublished doctoral dissertation, University of Vermont, Burlington, Vermont.

Harding, C. M., and G. W. Brooks. 1980. Longitudinal assessment for a cohort of chronic schizophrenics discharged twenty years ago. *Psychiatric Journal of the Unviersity of Ottawa* 5: 274–78.

Harding, C. M., G. W. Brooks, T. Ashikaga, J. S. Strauss, and P. D. Landerl. In press. Aging and social functioning in once-chronic schizophrenic patients 21–58 years after first admission: The Vermont story. In G. Hudgins and N. Miller (Eds.), *Schizophrenia, paranoia and schizophreniform disorders in later life.* New York: Guilford Press.

Harding, C. M. and J. S. Strauss. In press. The course of schizophrenia: An evolving concept. In M. Alpert (Ed.), *Controversies in schizophrenic changes and constancies.* New York: Guilford Press.

Hesse, M. 1980. *Revolutions and reconstructions in the philosophy of science.* Bloomington: Indiana University Press.

Huber, G., G. Gross, R. Schutter, and M. Linz. 1980. Longitudinal studies of schizophrenic patients. *Schizophrenia Bulletin,* 6: 592–605.

Kantor, J. R. 1926. *Principles of psychology,* vol. 2. Granville, Ohio: Principia Press.

Kantor, J. R. 1953. *The logic of modern science.* Granville, Ohio: Principia Press.

Kantor, J. R. 1959. *Interbehavioral psychology.* Granville, Ohio: Principia Press.

Kantor, J. R. 1963. *The scientific evolution of psychology,* vol. 1. Granville, Ohio: Principia Press.

Lamb, H. R., and V. Goertzel. 1977. The long-term patient in the era of community treatment. *Archives of General Psychiatry,* 34: 679–82.

Lincoln, Y. S., and E. G. Guba. 1985. *Naturalistic inquiry.* Beverly Hills, Calif.: Sage.

Moore, G., (Ed.) 1983. *Beyond method: Strategies for social research.* Beverly Hills, Calif.: Sage.

Morgan, G. I. 1983. Rethinking corporate strategy: A cybernetic perspective. *Human Relations* 36: 345–60.

Mountjoy, P. T. 1974. Methodological note: The United States Patent Office as a source of historical documents. *Journal of the History of the Behavioral Sciences* 10: 119–20.

Mountjoy, P. T. and G. W. Sears. 1971. Methodological note: Obtaining rare, out-of-print English language books printed before 1700. *Journal of the History of the Behavioral Sciences* 7: 75–76.

Stephens, J. H. 1978. Long-term prognosis and followup in schizophrenia. *Schizophrenia Bulletin* 4: 25–47.

Stephens, J. H., C. Astrup, and J. C. Mangrum. 1966. Prognostic factors in recovered and deteriorated schizophrenics. *American Journal of Psychiatry* 122: 1116–21.

Strauss, J. S. and W. T. Carpenter, Jr. 1974a. Characteristic symptoms and outcome of schizophrenia. *Archives of General Psychiatry* 30: 429–34.

Strauss, J. S. and W. T. Carpenter, Jr. 1974b. The prediction of outcome in schizophrenia. *Archives of General Psychiatry* 31: 37–42.

Strauss, J. S. and W. T. Carpenter, Jr. 1981. *Schizophrenia*. New York: Plenum.

Strauss, J. S., and W. Glazer. 1982. Treatment of the so-called chronically psychiatrically ill. *Current Psychiatric Therapies* 21: 207–17.

Strauss, J. S., and H. Hafez. 1981. Clinical questions and "real" research. *American Journal of Psychiatry* 138: 1592–97.

Strauss, J. S., H. Hafez, P. Lieberman, and C. M. Harding. 1985. The course of psychiatric disorder, III: Longitudinal principles. *American Journal of Psychiatry* 142: 289–96.

Strauss, J. S., L. Loevsky, W. Glazer, and P. Leaf. 1981. Organizing the complexities of schizophrenia. *Journal of Nervous and Mental Disease* 169: 120–26.

Tsuang, M. T. 1982. Long-term outcome in schizophrenia. *Trends in Neuroscience* 5: 203–7.

Tsuang, M. T. and M. Dempsey. 1979. Long-term outcome of major psychoses II. *Archives of General Psychiatry* 36: 1302–4.

Tsuang. M. T., R. F. Woolson, and J. A. Fleming. 1979. Long-term outcome of major psychoses I. *Archives of General Psychiatry* 36: 1295–1301.

Tsuang, M. T., R. F. Woolson, and J. C. Simpson. 1980. The Iowa structured psychiatric interview. *Acta Psychiatrica Scandinavica, Supplementum, 283*, vol. 62.

Tuma, A. H., P. R. May, C. Yale, and A. B. Forsythe. 1978. Therapist characteristics and the outcome of treatment in schizophrenia. *Archives of General Psychiatry* 35: 81–85.

Vaillant, G. E. 1978. A 10-year followup of remitting schizophrenics. *Schizophrenia Bulletin* 4: 78–85.

Vaughan, C. E., and J. P. Leff. 1976. The influence of family and social factors on the course of psychiatric illness. *British Journal of Psychiatry* 129: 125–37.

Woolson, R. F., M. T. Tsuang, and L. R. Urban. 1980. Data management in an epidemiological study: Experiences from the Iowa 500 field follow-up and family study. *Methods of Information in Medicine* 19: 37–41.

14

Value of "New Ideas"

Douglas H. Ruben and Dennis J. Delprato

In this final chapter we attempt to answer the basic question facing this volume. Why are these "new ideas" a value to clinical science and particularly to the application of psychological knowledge? After reading through each chapter, it becomes immediately apparent that psychology is one among the many related clinical disciplines (social work, counseling, psychiatry, nursing, and so on) that are interdisciplinary. For example, psychologists specializing in the study of pediatric disorders draw heavily upon the data base of medical and socioecological research to answer even the most elementary questions about etiology. Treatment of enuresis is a case in point. Typically the assessment of nocturnal or diurnal wetting begins by exhausting possible medical reasons for improper bladder control. Once urologic obstructions or diseases are ruled out, questions are appropriate regarding dynamics of familial interaction, maladaptive behavioral patterns and related functional difficulties. Completion of the assessment and then treatment depends primarily on knowledge of factors beyond the usual scope of psychological clinical inquiry.

To a growing number of psychologists, expansion of the modern clinical approach to other disciplines represents an exciting departure from traditional ways. Recently there have been trends in behavioral psychology exactly in this direction, of enlarging the operant/respondent paradigm to include scientifically inferred variables such as "sensory integration" (for example, behavioral neurology) and "developmental span" (behavioral pediatrics). Whether behaviorism in its most radical form is too shallow or behavioral therapists themselves find it too boring or mechanistic really does not motivate undertakings for the broader perspective. What really seems to be the cause for alarm is increasing recognition that, *on a scientific level*, behavioral principles and theories omit critical systems of analysis similar to those of all the established natural sciences. Absent is all concern with such matters as multiple causality including variables historically as well as potentially interrelated in the client's (human organism's) development over time. Understanding contingencies of reinforcement (and punishment) certainly is a start. But how about the origins of the reinforcers? What about the demographic, epidemiologic, or idiographic dictates in the culture—was the client rich or poor and did he come from a large or small community? Questions such as these are only tangentially addressed by the theoretical frameworks of behavioral practitioners and of clinicians generally.

To illustrate further the much needed interrelationship of field or systems concepts, consider some unpleasant pragmatics of behavioral therapy in the private sector. Referrals made to behavioral practitioners generally center on a limited number of childhood or adult disorders considered entirely symptomatic, for example, disruptive classroom behavior. If viewed and treated based on symptoms alone, practitioners might present M & M's on a differential reinforcement schedule for on-task sitting. However, little has been gained as far as constructive changes in the client's environment; important questions about the field remain unanswered. Is the problem that of the child or of the teacher? Do other children disrupt the class or is the problem individualistic? More important, is the client's disruptive behavior endemic to the classroom, *that classroom*, or does it reappear in multiple classes, in multiple schools, or in multiple settings? Answers to these questions first call upon the labor-intensive efforts of the practitioner to know more about the client, his field history (or reactional biography), and the involvement of additional variables.

A second problem is when behavioral practitioners encounter other professionals who are not supportive of behavioral viewpoints. Traditional psychotherapists, for example, often view the behavioral practitioner as simplistic in treatment approach and highly resistant to ideas apart from operational functions of the antecedent, behavior, and consequence. Nonpsychologists and nonmental health professionals may also share this viewpoint whether or not they subscribe to the dynamic explanation of problem resolution. A difference in viewpoint directly discourages a referral, consultation, or interaction with behavioral practitioners on such matters as social policy (e.g., licensing laws, peer-review committees, political campaigns), human service networks (e.g., HMOs, EAPs), and community issues (e.g., racism, fertility-mortality rates, unemployment). Problems with broad and specific consequences for individuals and society are routed to nonbehavioral specialists largely because of unfavorable perceptions of what a behaviorist knows or does not know.

Overcoming the barriers to effective intercourse between behaviorally and nonbehaviorally trained professionals does not begin, as many behaviorists contend, by educating colleagues in the philosophy and psychology of Watson, Skinner, or even Kantor. While there is room for education among all professionals, simply imposing one viewpoint (behaviorism) upon another viewpoint, one set of technical jargon upon another set of technical jargon, is missing the basic point. There is the *underlying science of psychology* to consider; particulars of events, constructs, and interactions among historical, current, and future fields of individual behavior transcend salient differences in each discipline. Consider an analysis of bulimia. Behaviorally the pattern involves purging and binging; the discipline of dentistry warns us that stomach juices (acids) decay tooth enamel; the discipline of medicine points out that reliance on laxatives may form a physical dependency. On the surface these three perspectives seem unrelated other than categorically referring to bulimia. Viewed interbehaviorally, however, each perspective is not mutually exclusive but rather is *interdependent* in that the full scientific analysis of bulimia can result only when all three (plus additional) perspectives combine together.

That is the purpose of "new ideas." This volume directly introduced specific pathways by which a more solid scientific approach to human behavior can be applied across disciplines. Knowledge of and experience in this emerging form of interdisciplinary psychology is obtained, first, through an atmosphere of open-minded evaluation and discussion. Second, it requires that behavioral practitioners be informed about the assumptions, methods, and goals of alternative approaches. Finally, exposure to eclectic study in an objective manner should be sure to include a strong understanding of natural sciences. The result can be practitioners with greater compatibility among nonbehavioral practitioners and who distinctly seek out professionals in related fields. Although a seemingly tedious task, it is much the same approach medical science took earlier in the century when it crossed that "fine line" into social science. Now the time has come for the social scientist, the mental health practitioner, to return the favor.

Index

ABA. *See* Applied behavior analysis

Abnormal personalities. *See* Psychopathology

Agras, W. S., 80

Alexander, J. F., 152

Alternating personalities, 47, 48

Amnesia, 47–48

Antisocial personalities, 44; case study, 24–25; in children, 54, 59, 60–61, 62–69, 70

Anxious personalities, 42

Applied behavior analysis (ABA), 53–54, 56, 137; behavioral contrast, 59; behavioral systems strategy, 60; behavior regulation, 58; child prosocial behaviors, 56, 57; matching laws, 60; molar assessment, 60, 63, 74; molecular assessment, 60, 63, 74; reinforcement, 53; response cluster, 57; response concept, 53, 54, 57–58; response covariation, 54, 56, 57–58; setting factors, 59, 60; side effects, 57; stimulus concept, 53–54, 58–60; three-term operant principle, 53–54, 56–57, 58, 59. *See also* TEAB

Ashby, W. R., 82

Assertiveness Skills Training Groups (ASTGs), 108–9, 110, 111, 112

Assertiveness training, 107–17; acquisition, 107, 110, 112, 116; behavioral methods, 107; causality, 111; cognitive methods, 107; dimensions of assertiveness, 112; for domestic violence victims, 112; environment interactions, 113, 116–17; failures in, 110, 116; follow-up, 107, 116; functional descriptions, 109–11, 112, 116; generalization, 112–14, 116; goals, 115; interbehavioral potential, 111; intrapsychic dynamics, 108, 109, 116; learning interactions, 110–11; maintenance, 107, 116; objectives, 115; physical descriptions, 108–9, 112; stimulus generalization, 112, 113; training model, 114–16; voice-control skills, 112

ASTGs. (Assertiveness Skills Training Groups), 108–9, 110, 111, 112

Autism, 171–72

Bachrac, Leona, 203

Baer, D. M., 168

Barker, R. G., 163
Beck Depression Inventory, 67
Behavioral ecological psychology, 163
Behavioral medicine. *See* Interbehavioral
   medicine
Behavioral parent training, 159, 160–62;
   assumptions, 160–61; extradyadic vari-
   ables, 161–62, 164, 172; studies, 161;
   three-term contingency, 172; training
   groups, 161
Behavioral psychology, 16, 209–11
Behavior analysis. *See* Applied behavior
   analysis (ABA); TEAB
Behavior modification, 74, 80, 81, 90–
   91, 102, 110, 137; with develop-
   mentally disabled (DD), 24, 180–81
Behavior Problem Checklist, 61
Bennet, W., 120
Bentley, A. F., 14–16
Berkson, G., 182
Binet, A., 37
Biofeedback, 80, 90–91
Birmingham (Michigan) YMCA. *See*
   Health Life Program (HLP)
Blanchard, E. B., 80
Bleuler, Eugen, 201
Brooks, G. W., 193
Brownell, K. D., 120
Bulimia, 211

Cancer, 83
Carnegie, Dale, 108
Catatonic personalities, 44
Child abuse, 70, 171
Child Behavior Checklist, 61, 67
Child-parent interbehavior. *See* Child
   psychology; Interbehavioral medicine,
   child-parent study
Child psychology, 53, 60–75; academic
   response study, 55; antisocial behaviors, 54, 59, 60–61, 62–69, 70; assessment of parents, 61; assessment self-
   reports, 61, 64, 65–66, 67–69, 71–72,
   73; autism study, 171–72; aversive parental actions, 58–59, 60, 61–62, 63,
   65–66, 70–74, 83; Beck Depression
   Inventory, 67; Behavior Problem
   Checklist, 61; child abuse, 70, 171;

Child Behavior Checklist, 61, 67; class
   comparisons, 68–69; class description,
   63, 64; clinical assessment, 63–69;
   coercive cycles study, 171; Connors
   Parent Rating Scale, 61; covertly oppositional behaviors, 64, 68; dependency
   behaviors, 60, 61, 70; Dyadic Adjustment Scale, 172; enuresis, 209; Family
   Environment Scale, 172; insular parent
   study, 170–71; marital relations and,
   53; MMPI, 172; molar responses, 63,
   64, 67, 68, 69, 70; molecular responses, 63, 64, 67, 68, 71; overtly
   oppositional behaviors, 64, 67–68; parent depression, 63, 65–66, 68, 70; parent enhancement therapy, 171; parent
   irritability characteristic, 65; parent reaction to behaviors, 65, 67–69; response classes, 62–63; response
   cluster, 70; response conceptions, 63–
   66, 68; response covariatons, 62;
   schizophrenic movement study, 58;
   sharing behavior study, 55–56, 59, 66;
   social smiling study, 56, 57; solitary
   play behavior, 54, 63, 70; stealing behaviors, 64; stimulus-class model, 61–
   62; stimulus conceptions, 66–67, 68–
   69. *See also* Applied behavior analysis
   (ABA); Behavioral parent training; Developmentally disabled (DD); Interbehavioral medicine, child-parent study;
   TEAB
Child psychology, clinical intervention,
   69–74; clinician, 74–75; contingency
   management, 69–71, 73, 74–75; contracting, 69; ignoring, 63, 69; indirect
   effects, 69; for keystone responses,
   70–71; mand review, 73; material rewards, 69; parent training, 69; praise,
   69, 71; response-cost, 63; for sequential patterns, 69–70; stimulus-class
   modifications, 71–74; surveillance
   training, 69; three-term operant contingency, 69; time-out contingency, 62,
   63, 69–70, 71
Clinical psychology, 7–8, 18–20; doctoral
   program in, 26–27; medical practice
   and, 8, 26; personal observations

about, 23–24; research methodology, 9–21, 25; theory and, 17–18

Clinician, 74–75, 183–85, 189

Comprehensive Drug Abuse Prevention and Control Act of 1970, 146

Compulsive personalities, 45–46

Connors Parent Rating Scale, 61

Conversion reactions, 39–40, 47–48

Criminal personalities, 41. *See also* Legal deviance

Cybernetic control theory, 82

da Vinci, Leonardo, 10

Defective personalities, 42, 43–46; catatonic personalities, 44; compulsive personalities, 45–46; delinquent personalities, 43–44; hypochondrial personalities, 45; inhibitive personalities, 46; paranoid personalities, 44; schizophrenic personalities, 44–45; vacillating personalities, 46

Degenerating personalities, 42, 48–49; paretic personalities, 49; senile personalities, 48–49

Delinquent personalities, 43–44. *See also* Legal deviance

Delprato, Dennis J., 83–84, 122–23

Delusions, 44

Depressive personalities, 46–47

Developmentally disabled (DD), 8, 43, 179–89; assessment of, 183–84, 187, 188; behavior compliance, 185, 186; behavior modification, 24, 280–81; chemical treatment for, 181, 186; clinician role, 183–85, 189; definition of, 181; documentation of intervention procedures, 188; generalization, 185, 186; hand-washing case study, 186–88; impact on family, 161–62, 171, 172, 181; inappropriate behavior of, 166, 180, 183, 184–85; institutional care of, 180; intelligence measurements, 181, 183–84; interbehavioral history, 185; interdisciplinary treatment team, 183, 184; testing of, 183–84; treatment of, 181, 183, 184–85, 188

Developmentally disabled (DD) children, parent-training, 159–72, 181–82; assessment of research studies, 169–70; autism study, 171–72; behavioral parent training, 159, 160–62; child abuse study, 171; coercive cycles study, 171; component analysis, 167–68; control groups, 167; data collection, 164, 168; Dyadic Adjustment Scale, 172; extradyadic variables, 161–62, 164, 172; Family Environment Scale, 172; follow-up, 169; generalization, 164, 168–69; impact on family, 161–62, 171, 172; insular parent study, 170–71; limitations of research studies, 164, 165, 172; maintenance, 164, 169; MMPI, 172; parent characteristics, 164, 166; parent enhancement therapy, 171; parent trainers, 164, 166; research review, 164–70; sample size of research studies, 164, 165; setting factors, 171; subjects of research studies, 164, 165; three-term contingency, 160, 172; training obstacles, 168; training procedures, 164, 167–68; training side-effects, 168–69

Dewey, J., 14–16

Differential reinforcement, 25

Differential reinforcement of alternative behavior (DRA), 180

Differential reinforcement of zero-based behavior (DRO), 180

Disintegrating personalities, 43, 46–47, 50; depressive personalities, 46–47; manic personalities, 46–47

Disorganized personalities, 42, 49

Dissociated personalities, 42, 47–48, 50–51; conversion reactions, 39–40, 47–48; multiple personalities, 47, 48; reactive dissociation, 47

Domestic violence, 112

DRA (differential reinforcement of alternative behavior), 180

DRO (differential reinforcement of zero-based behavior), 180

Drug abuse, legal deviance and, 144–47

Dyadic Adjustment Scale, 172

Education programs, 31, 32–34

Einstein, A., 82

Employment programs, 30–31
Enuresis, 209
Epileptic seizures, 46
Experimental analysis of behavior. *See* TEAB
Extinction procedures, 182

Factor theory, 95, 98
Family. *See* Child psychology; Developmentally disabled (DD); Legal deviance
Family Environment Scale, 172
Ferster, C., 54
Field psychology. *See* Clinical psychology
Fields. *See* Psychological fields
Freedman, J. L., 142
Freud, Sigmund, 42, 45
Fuller, P. R., 120

Galton, Francis, 37
Generalization, 112, 113, 168; in assertiveness training, 112–14, 116; in developmentally disabled (DD), 164, 168–69, 185, 186; in legal deviance, 148, 149–50; stimulus-control perspective, 150
Global Assessment Scale, 198, 199
Guba, E. G., 195, 196, 204
Gurin, J., 120
Guthrie, E., 160

Handicapped. *See* Developmentally disabled (DD)
Hanson, N. R., 12, 14, 15
Harding, C. M., 193, 196
Healthy Life Program (HLP), 132–34; clients, 132; fitness evaluation, 133, 134; follow-up, 134; helping agents, 133; meetings, 132–33, 134; orientation, 132; outcome data, 134; record-keeping, 133, 134; staff, 132. *See also* Obesity and Risk Factor Program (ORFP); Obesity management
Hermeneutics, 104
Hesse, Mary, 194–95
Hippocrates, 46
HLP. *See* Healthy Life Program

Hypochondrial personalities, 45
Hysterical personalities, 39–40, 47–48

Inappropriate behavior, 38; of developmentally disabled (DD), 166, 180, 183, 184–85
Infeld, L., 82
Information theory analyses, 152
Inhibitive personalities, 46
Intergrated-field perspective. *See* Psychological fields
Interbehavioral medicine, 79–91; behavior modification, 80, 81, 90–91; for cancer patients, 83; conceptual organization, 80–84; evolutional postulate, 122, 123; experimental analysis of behavior, 81, 90–91; field postulate, 122, 123; goal postulate, 123; history of, 79–80, 90–91; holistic postulate, 122; interbehavioral field theory, 82–83, 91; interdisciplinary postulate, 122, 123; postulates, 83–84, 122–23; systems theory, 82, 91; tactical postulate, 122–23
Interbehavioral medicine, child-parent study, 84–91; agitation behavior, 85, 86, 87–89; analytical units, 85; attachment behavior, 85, 89; autodependence, 86, 87, 88; behavioral inertia, 86; cross-dependence, 86–87, 88, 89–90; data collection, 85; distracting behavior, 85; distress behavior, 85, 86, 87–89; dominance, 86, 87; existing research, 84; General Linear Model, 86; ignoring behavior, 85; informing behavior, 85; N-behavior system, 89–91; reassuring behavior, 85, 87; research methodology, 85–91; research setting, 85; sampling interval, 85–86; sequential patterns, 86, 88; subjects, 85
Interbehavioral psychology, 3–8, 18–21, 82–83, 91, 108, 137, 139, 153, 162–63, 182; clinician, 74–75, 183–85, 189; comparison to existing frameworks, 163; interbehavioral history, 139–40, 144, 185; medium of contact, 19; molar assessment, 163; as natural science, 3–4; observations, 3, 4, 12–

14, 18, 19, 20; psychological field components, 4–6, 19, 108, 113, 150–51, 179, 194; reified constructs, 141–42; setting factors, 19–20, 33, 59, 60, 144–50, 162–63

Interbehavioral Psychology (Kantor), 194

Iowa Structured Psychiatric Interview, 197

Kantor, J. R., 37–51, 56, 59, 74, 82–83, 91, 100, 104, 108, 139, 159–60, 162–63, 170, 172, 179, 183, 192, 193, 193–94, 196, 204, 205

Kohut, H., 103

Kraeplin, Emil, 201

Kuhn, T. S., 10–11, 15, 16

Lag sequential analyses, 152

Lazarus, A., 108

Learning theory, 74, 108, 110–11, 112, 113, 114, 116, 160; interbehavioral potentials, 111; learning interactions, 111

Legal deviance, 32, 137–53; contextual perspective, 138–39; criminal thinking patterns, 141; from crowding, 142–43; drug-crime research, 144–45; drug laws and social policy, 144, 145–47; drugs in violent crime, 144, 145, 146; drug treatment programs, 145; environmental setting factors, 147–50; generalization, 148, 149–50; impact on family, 149, 151–52; information theory analyses, 152; interbehavioral history, 139–40, 141, 142, 143, 147; interdisciplinary research, 148–49; intervention procedures, 138–39, 149, 151, 152, 153; lag sequential analyses, 152; maintenance, 148, 149–50; from male XYY genotype, 140–41; Markov chain analyses, 152; matching law, 149; from mental and biological processes, 140, 141–42; from mental and biological traits, 140–41; organismic setting factors, 144–47, 150; physical-chemical setting factors, 147; psychological fields, 151–52; from situationism, 140, 142–43; social-cultural

setting factors, 147–48; stealing behaviors, 64; stimulus-control perspective of generalization, 150; vandalism study, 148

Lincoln Y. S., 195, 196, 204

Lindsley, O., 54

Linguistic evolution, 6–7

Living systems theory, 82

Logic of Modern Science (Kantor), 193

McGlynn, F. D., 83–84, 122–23

Maintenance, 169; in assertiveness training, 107, 116; in developmentally disabled (DD), 164, 169; in legal deviance, 148, 149–50; in obesity management, 127–28

Management assertiveness training, 114–16; analysis, 116; follow-up, 115–16; goals, 115; objectives, 115; structure, 115, 116

Management development program, 28–29

Mand review, 73

Manic personalities, 46–47

Markov chain analyses, 152

Matching law, 59–60, 149

Mentally disturbed. *See* Psychopathology; Public mental health policy

Meyer, Adolph, 201

Miller, J. G., 82

Minuchin, S., 181

MMPI, 172

Morgan, Gareth, 204

Multiple personalities, 47, 48

Nondirective therapy, 24–25

Obesity and Risk Factor Program (ORFP), 123–31, 132, 135; advanced maintenance, 128; client data system, 124, 126, 128–29; clients, 124; continued fasting, 127; early fasting, 126–27; early maintenance, 127–28; family session, 126; imaginary fast, 126; intermediate maintenance, 128; life-style assessment, 124; physical examinations, 126; prefasting, 124, 126; record review, 126; refeeding process, 127;

risk-factor review, 128; staff, 124; staff data system, 129–31; summary studies, 131. *See also* Healthy Life Program (HLP); Obesity management

Obesity management, 119–35; behavioral approach, 119; evolutional postulate, 122, 123; field-factor approach, 120–22; field postulate, 122, 123; goal postulate, 123; holistic postulate, 122; interdisciplinary postulate, 122, 123; program guidelines, 122–23; set-point theory, 119–20; tactical postulate, 122–23. *See also* Healthy Life Program (HLP); Obesity and Risk Factor Program (ORFP)

Observations, 3, 4, 12–14, 18, 19, 20; theory-laden seeing, 14, 17

Operant learning theory. *See* Learning theory

Operant psychology. *See* Behavior modification

ORFP. *See* Obesity and Risk Factor Program

Orlando (Woolf), 96, 104

Paradigms, 10–16; interaction, 15–16; observation, 12–14; paradigm shift, 11–12; self-action, 14–15, 16; transaction, 16

Paranoid personalities, 44

Parent-child interrelationship. *See* Child psychology

Parent training. *See* Behavioral parent training; Developmentally disabled (DD) children, parent-training

Paretic personalities, 49

Parloff's law, 102, 103

Pathological personalities, 8, 40, 42–50; catatonic personalities, 44; compulsive personalities, 45–46; conversion reactions, 47–48; defective personalities, 42, 43–46; degenerating personalities, 42, 48–49; delinquent personalities, 43–44; depressive personalities, 46–47; disintegrating personalities, 42, 46–47, 50; disorganized personalities, 42, 49; dissociated personalities, 42, 47–48, 50–51; hypochondrial personalities, 45;

inhibitive personalities, 46; manic personalities, 46–47; multiple personalities, 47, 48; paranoid personalities, 44; paretic personalities, 49; reactive dissociation, 47; schizophrenic personalities, 44–45; senile personalities, 48–49; traumatic personalities, 42, 49–50; undeveloped personalities, 42, 43, 50; vacillating personalities, 46. *See also* Public mental health policy

Pattens of Discovery (Hanson), 12, 14

Patterson, G. R., 152, 181–82

Pearson, Karl, 15

Pennick, S. B., 119

Perlin's law, 102, 103

Personality. *See* Psychological personality

Pigeon pecking study, 56–57

Pomerleau, O. F., 80, 81

Popper, K. R., 102

Posttraumatic stress reactions, 49

Principles of Psychology (Kantor), 192

Psychiatrist's Global Rating of Illness Scale, 199

Psychodynamics, 61

Psychological complaints, 7–8; pathological behavior, 8; severity of, 7; type of, 7; unadaptable behavior, 8; unusual behavior, 7. *See also specific complaint*

Psychological fields, 4–6, 19, 108, 113, 150–51, 179, 194; adaptations, 4; definite field origins, 4; functions, 6; individual evolution, 4; interbehaviors, 4–6, 7, 18, 25, 26, 113, 116–17; psychological personality, 4–6; stimulus objects, 6, 19

Psychological personality, 4–6; communal traits, 5; idiosyncratic traits, 5–6, 7, 37–38, 50; interbehaviors, 4–6, 7, 18, 25, 26, 113, 116–17; maturation stages, 5, 7; personality evolution, 5–6; psychological evolution, 6–7

Psychopathology, 37–51; anxious personalities, 42; behavior equipment, 38; catatonic personalities, 44; classification of abnormality, 40–51; compulsive personalities, 45–46; conversion reactions, 47–48; criminal personalities, 41; criteria of abnormality, 38–40; defective personalities, 42, 43–46; degenerating personalities, 42, 48–49; delinquent personalities, 43–44; depressive personalities, 46–47; disintegrating personalities, 42, 46–47, 50; disorganized personalities, 42, 49; dissociated personalities, 42, 47–48, 50–51; heredity factors, 43; hypochondrial personalities, 45; immediate behavior surroundings, 39; inappropriate behavior, 38; inhibitive personalities, 46; interbehavioral history, 38–39; manic personalities, 46; multiple personalities, 47, 48; paranoid personalities, 44; paretic personalities, 49; pathological personalities, 40, 42–50; reaction system defects, 39–40, 43; reactive dissociation, 47; schizophrenic personalities, 44–45; senile personalities, 48–49; traumatic personalities, 42, 49–50; unadaptable personalities, 40, 41, 50; undeveloped personalities, 42, 43, 50; unusual personalities, 40–41, 50; vacillating personalities, 46. *See also* Public mental health policy

Psychophysical psychology, 15

Public mental health policy, 191–206; analysis of existing research, 194–96; Bonn study, 197; Boston study, 199; Brooklyn study, 198–99; chronicity study, 203–4; client profile, 205–6; client recovery, 204; client self-control techniques, 204; client treatment procedures, 204–5; community living *vs.* institutionalization, 205; Development Model, 204–5; effective program design principles, 203; field models, 203–5; Global Assessment Scale, 198, 199; Iowa 500 study, 197; Iowa Structured Psychiatric Interview, 197; Lausanne study, 197–98; longitudinal studies, 192–93, 196, 197–200, 205; Manhattan hotel study, 202; married *vs.* unmarried clients, 197, 203; Massachusetts Mental Health Center study, 200, 201; Ponoka study, 199; predicting good outcome, 200–203; primary studies, 196–200; program evaluations,

192–94; Psychiatrist's Global Rating of Illness Scale, 199; qualitative approach, 203; research methods, 193–94; San Mateo study, 202–3; significant others studies, 202; Supplemental Security Income (SSI) study, 202–3; therapist characteristics study; Vermont Longitudinal Research Project, 198; WHO (World Health Organization) International Pilot Study of Schizophrenia, 201–2. *See also* Pathological personalities; Psychopathology

Punishment procedures, 182

Q methodology, 95–104; analyst/patient intersubjectivity study, 102–3; behavioral segment, 95–96, 99–100; behavior modification, 102; concourse, 96, 97, 99; condition of instruction, 100, 101; factor arrays, 101–2; factor loading, 103; factor structure, 101, 104; formalization, 99–101; intersubjectivity, 102–3; Parloff's law, 102, 103; Perlin's law, 102, 104; Q-sample, 97, 99, 101; Q-sort, 97–100, 101, 104; Roger's law, 103; self-reference statements, 96, 99, 104; tea obsession study, 97–99, 101–2, 104; theory of concourse, 97; theory of self, 96–97; transference situation, 103; vital sign, 99, 103, 104

Quantum theory, 104

Reactive dissociation, 47

Research methodology, 9–21; analysis of existing studies, 194–96; for child psychology, 61, 67; crude data, 193; cultural sources, 193–94; for developmentally disabled (DD) studies, 172; direct observation, 193; historico-critical level, 194; identification of primary studies, 196; impact of values on studies, 195; instrumental observation, 193; interaction, 15–16, 17, 18; investigator's values, 195, 196, 204; for legal deviance studies, 152; longitudinal studies, 192–93; for mental health studies, 197, 198, 199; observation,

17, 18; operations, 193; products, 193; remote observation, 193–94, 205; self-action, 14–15, 16, 17, 18, 19; tertiary scientific level, 194; theory, 10, 16–21; thing and event matrix, 193, 194, 196; transaction, 16, 17; transforming contacts, 193

Response decrement procedures, 182

Retardation. *See* Developmentally disabled (DD)

Risk-factor management. *See* Healthy Life Program (HLP); Obesity and Risk Factor Program (ORFP); Obesity management

Roges's law, 103

Salter, A., 108

Samenow, S. E., 141

Schizophrenia, 44–45, 58, 197–200, 205; course of, 204; predicting good outcome, 200–203; WHO (World Health Organization) International Pilot Study of Schizophrenia, 201–2. *See also* Public mental health policy

Schwartz, G. E., 82

Scibak, J. W., 180

Secondary gain, 45

Senile personalities, 48–49

Set-point theory, 119–20

Setting factors, 19–20, 33, 59, 60, 144–50, 162–63, 171; drugs as, 144–47; environmental, 144, 147, 162; organismic, 144, 147, 150, 162; physical-chemical, 147; social-cultural, 147–48

Shakespeare, William, 16

Simon, T., 37

Skinner, B. F., 20, 56, 57, 58, 110, 160, 163

Space program, 29–30

Spearman, Charles, 95, 101

Staddon, J. E. R., 120

Stimulus-response psychology, 15, 19

Stokes, T. F., 168

Strauss, J. S., 196

The Structure of Scientific Revolutions (Kuhn), 10–11

Stunkard, A. J., 119, 123–24

Suicide, 47

Sullivan, Harry Stack, 18

Systems theory, 82, 91

TEAB (The Experimental Analysis of Behavior), 54–55, 56, 81, 90–91; behavioral contrast, 55; behavior-environment experiences, 55, 56; matching laws, 59–60; molar assessment, 55; pigeon pecking study, 56–57; reinforcement, 55; response units, 54–55, 56, 58; stimulus units, 55–56; superstitious stimulus control, 55, 59. *See also* Applied behavior analysis (ABA)

Theory, 10, 16–21; clinical psychology and, 17–18; data and construct relationship, 20–21; interaction, 17, 18; revolutions in, 16; self-action, 17, 18; transaction, 17

Three-term contingency, 53–54, 56–57, 58, 59, 160, 163, 172

Timberlake, W., 58

Traumatic personalities, 42, 49–50

Tsuang, M. T., 196

Unadaptable personalities, 8, 40, 41, 50

Undeveloped personalities, 42, 43, 50

Unusual personalities, 7, 40–41, 50

Vacillating personalities, 46

Vandalism study, 148

von Bertalanffy, L., 82

Wahler, R. G., 163

Watson, J., 16

Wayne State University. *See* Obesity and Risk Factor Program (ORFP)

Whitman, T. L., 180

Willems, E. P., 57

Williams, C., 161

Wolpe, J., 108

Woodger, J. H., 9–10

Woolf, Virginia, 96–97, 98, 104

YMCA. *See* Healthy Life Program (HLP)

Yochelson, S., 141

About the Editors and Contributors

DONNA M. CONE is Associate Director of the Rhode Island State Department of Mental Health, Retardation, and Hospitals and an Adjunct Associate Professor of Psychology at the University of Rhode Island. She serves on the Board of Editors of *The Psychological Record* and *The Interbehaviorist*. Her areas of specialty include biological psychology, evaluation research, and the history of the behavioral sciences.

EDWIN W. COOK III is Assistant Professor in the Department of Psychology at the University of Alabama at Birmingham. His research interests include the psychophysiology of emotion, human preparedness, and behavioral medicine.

LYNNE A. DAURELLE is psychologist at Firecrest School for the developmentally disabled and a doctoral candidate in clinical psychology and mental retardation in the Department of Psychology and Human Development at George Peabody College of Vanderbilt University. Her clinical and research interests include parent training with families of develomentally disabled persons, systems maintenance in institutional programming, and staff management issues.

DENNIS J. DELPRATO is Professor of Psychology at Eastern Michigan University where he is coordinator of the Clinical Behaviorial Program. He has published articles and chapters in both basic and clinic-applied science and is interested in bridging the gap that currently exists between the two areas.

JAMES J. FOX is Assistant Professor in the Department of Special Education and a research scientist in Mental Retardation and Human Development, George

Peabody College of Vanderbilt University. His research interests include the social development of children with mental retardation and behavior disorders, and parent training.

PAUL R. FULLER is a clinical psychologist and industrial consultant, as well as Professor at Muskegan College. He has pioneered the application of behavioral and interbehavioral psychology in clinical, school, organizational, engineering, and space psychology. He was particularly active in the science of Manned Space Systems, education, and research, and has taught at over a dozen colleges and universities.

PAUL E. GREENBAUM is Research Fellow in the Department of Clinical Psychology at the University of Florida. His research interests include children's fear and disruption to medical treatment, interpersonal behavior, and the communication of emotion and health psychology.

DELLA M. HANN is Assistant Professor at Louisiana State University at New Orleans. She is best known for her work on mother-infant relationships.

MICHAEL J. HEMINGWAY maintains a private practice and currently is Behavior Analyst Consultant with the Florida Department of Health and Rehabilitative Services. He was formerly Program Consultant for the Michigan Department of Mental Health. His research interests include the application of behavioral principles to a wide spectrum of clinical concerns.

LISA M. JOHNSON is a doctoral student and NICHHD predoctoral trainee in the Department of Human Development at the University of Kansas. She has published, presented, and conducted research in the experimental analysis of behavior particularly related to schedule-induced behavior and behavioral pharmacology.

ANN P. KAISER (formerly Rogers-Warren) is Associate Professor in the Department of Special Education at George Peabody College of Vanderbilt University. She serves on the editorial boards of several journals, including *Education and Treatment of Children* and *Analysis and Intervention of Developmental Disabilities*, and is co-editor of *Teaching Functional Language* and *Ecological Perspectives in Behavior Analysis*.

J. R. KANTOR (1888–1984) spent the majority of his academic career in the Department of Psychology at Indiana University. His contributions to psychology and philosophy are numerous. Books on psychology include *Principles of Psychology* (2 vols.), *A Survey of the Science of Psychology*, *An Objective Psychology of Grammar*, *Psychological Linguistics*, *Problems of Physiological Psychology*, *An Outline of Social Psychology*, *Cultural Psychology*, *Interbe-*

havioral Psychology, and *The Scientific Evolution Psychology* (2 vols.). Books on philosophy include *Psychology and Logic* (2 vols.), *The Logic of Modern Science*, *Interbehavioral Philosophy*, and *Tragedy and the Event Continuum*.

ROBERT W. LUNDIN is William R. Kenan Professor of Psychology and Department Chairman at the University of the South. His many articles and books reflect his interest in behavioristic attitudes, in the history of psychology, and in the application of interbehavioral psychology to personality, including *An Objective Psychology of Music*, *Personality: An Experimental Approach*, *Principles of Psychopathology*, and *Theories and Systems of Psychology*.

F. DUDLEY McGLYNN is Professor in the Department of Community Dentistry and the Department of Clinical Psychology at the University of Florida. His research interests include fear and avoidance, bruxism and facial pain, and compliance with prescribed self-care regimens.

WILLIAM E. MACLEAN, JR. is Assistant Professor of Psychology and Human Development and Co-Director of the Behavioral Pediatrics Clinic at George Peabody College of Vanderbilt University. His clinical and research interests include disabled children, the stereotyped and self-injurious behaviors of mentally retarded children and adults, and general behavioral pediatrics.

EDWARD K. MORRIS is Professor in the Department of Human Development and Family Life at the University of Kansas and Editor of *The Behavior Analyst* and *The Interbehaviorist*. His research interests include theoretical and clinical expansion of concepts in criminology, juvenile delinquency, and child development. He is co-editor of *Behavioral Approaches to Crime and Delinquency: Application, Research and Theory*.

LYNDA K. POWELL is a doctoral student in the Department of Counseling Psychology at the University of Kansas. She has published, presented papers, and conducted research on social and organizational systems, professional development of women, and sex development. Her clinical work focuses on children and families.

N. H. PRONKO is Emeritus Professor at University of Wichita. After thirty years and some 30,000 students, he currently dedicates his time to writing projects. Among his major books are *Panorama of Psychology*, *Psychology from the Standpoint of an Interbehaviorist*, and *AI to Zeitgeist: A Guide for the Skeptical Psychologist* (Greenwood Press, forthcoming).

DOUGLAS H. RUBEN is clinical psychologist in private practice, management consultant, and adjunct instructor at several colleges and universities. He is the author or co-author of over fifteen books and numerous articles on the applications of behavior therapy and interbehavioral psychology, including *Progress in Assertiveness*, *Reassessment in Psychology: The Interbehavioral Alternative*, and *Fundamentals of Substance Abuse Counseling*.

MARILYN J. RUBEN is Administrator for the Michigan Department of Labor and Assistant to the Executive Director of the Commission for the Blind. She is co-author of two books on psychology, including *60 Seconds to Success* with D. H. Ruben.

MARY ANN SCAFASCI is clinical psychologist in community-based agencies serving developmentally disabled individuals. Her research interests include the referral network and interbehavioral methodology for problems of the mentally retarded.

WILLIAM STEPHENSON was Director at the Institute of Experimental Psychology at the University of Oxford, then Research Professor at the University of Missouri-Columbia, and lecturer at the University of Chicago and the University of Iowa. He is best known for his introduction of "Q Methodology" and research in communication theory. Influenced by Kantor, his publications reflect field thinking in clinical topics. He is the author of *The Study of Behavior: Q-Technique and its Methodology*, and various articles published in *Psychological Record*.

DALLAS W. STEVENSON (1956–1986) was most recently Director of Behavioral Medicine at the Obesity and Risk Factor Clinic at Wayne State University, and a doctoral student at Western Michigan University. He made accelerated progress in the interbehavioral approach to weight problems and in behavioral medicine, reflected by his published papers and presentations at professional meetings.

JAMES T. TODD is a doctoral student and NICHHD predoctoral trainee in the Department of Human Development at the University of Kansas. He has published, presented papers, and conducted research in the experimental analysis of behavior including topics on schedule-induced behavior, covert behavior, and ethology.

ROBERT G. WAHLER is Professor of Psychology at the University of Tennessee, Knoxville and actively involved in research of parent-child problems using behavioral assessment and methodology. He is best known for his pioneering advances to expand the boundaries of traditional applied behavioral analysis. He is co-editor of *Ecological Assessment of Child Problem Behaviors*, and his articles frequently appear in *Behavioral Assessment*, *Journal of Applied Behavior Analysis*, and *Behavior Therapy*.